HYPERTENSION AND PREGNANCY

HYPERTENSION AND PREGNANCY

JAY M. SULLIVAN, M.D.

Professor of Medicine
Chief, Division of Cardiovascular Diseases
University of Tennessee Center for the Health Sciences
Memphis, Tennessee

YEAR BOOK MEDICAL PUBLISHERS, INC.
Chicago

0 9 8 7 6 5 4 3 2 1

Library of Congress Cataloging in Publication Data

Sullivan, Jay M.
    Hypertension and pregnancy.

    Bibliography: p.
    Includes index.
    1. Hypertension in pregnancy.   I. Title.   [DNLM:
1. Hypertension—in pregnancy.   2. Pregnancy
Complications, Cardiovascular.   WQ 244 S949h]
RG580.H9S85   1986   618.3   85–14200
ISBN 0–8151–8615–0

Sponsoring Editor: James D. Ryan, Jr.
Manager, Copyediting Services: Frances M. Perveiler
Production Project Manager: Etta Worthington
Proofroom Supervisor: Shirley E. Taylor

To my wife, Suzanne, and children,
Elizabeth, Suzanne, and Christopher

PREFACE

THIS BOOK HAS BEEN written for those health care professionals who either take care of patients with essential or secondary hypertension who become pregnant or who treat pregnant patients who become hypertensive. It should also serve as a useful reference source for those investigating the pathogenesis of these disorders. While the etiologies of neither essential hypertension nor pregnancy-induced hypertension or preeclampsia have been uncovered, considerable new information about the pathophysiologic changes accompanying these conditions has emerged as the result of recent research efforts. It is now clear that all hypertensive patients who become pregnant are not completely characterized by the designation chronic hypertension, for not only are there distinct secondary causes of chronic hypertension that require specific treatment, there are also pathophysiologic subdivisions of essential hypertension that also have implications for management. Similarly, not all patients who develop hypertension during pregnancy have the same disease processes. In some, essential hypertension is becoming apparent during gestation and in others, a specific disease process related to pregnancy has emerged. Further, the recent introduction of several new antihypertensive agents necessitates additional informed decision making on the part of the clinician. It is hoped that this book will help clarify these distinctions and contribute to the care of women with elevated blood pressure.

JAY M. SULLIVAN, M.D.

CONTENTS

Preface vii

1 / Introduction 1

2 / Classification 3

3 / Regulation of the Circulation 9

4 / Circulatory Adjustments to Pregnancy 13

5 / Essential Hypertension: Etiologic Considerations 19
    Hemodynamics of Human Hypertension 19
    Sodium, the Kidney, and the Heart 26
    Activity of the Sympathetic Nervous System 33
    The Renin-Angiotensin-Aldosterone System 36
    Prostaglandins and the Kallikrein-Kinin System 42
    Vasodepressor Lipids 67
    Membrane Transport and Hypertension 68
    Comparison of Essential and Pregnancy-Induced
        Hypertension 71

6 / Pregnancy-Induced Hypertension: Etiologic Considerations . . . 73
    Impaired Uteroplacental Perfusion 74
    Cardiovascular Changes in Hypertensive Pregnancy 78
    Vascular Reactivity in Preeclampsia-Eclampsia 80
    Renal Changes in Hypertensive Pregnancy 82
    Endocrine Changes in Normal and Hypertensive Pregnancy . . 85
    Prostaglandins, the Kallikrein-Kinin System, and Pregnancy . . 89
    Hemostasis in Hypertensive Pregnancy 93
    Magnesium and Calcium 94
    Helminths and Preeclampsia 96
    The Immune Response and Preeclampsia 97

7 / Consequences of Elevated Blood Pressure 103
    Rationale for Treatment 106

8 / Consequences of Elevated Blood Pressure During
    Pregnancy 113
    Prognosis of Pregnancy-Induced Hypertension 116

9 / Goals of Antihypertensive Therapy 121

10 / Antihypertensive Management 123
    Considerations During Pregnancy 125

11 / Pathophysiologic Subdivisions of Essential Hypertension 147

12 / Management of Patients With Preeclampsia-Eclampsia 151

13 / Hypertensive Emergencies and Urgencies 157

14 / Pregnancy and Secondary Hypertension 161
    Hypertension Secondary to Renal Disease 161
    Hypertension Secondary to Adrenal Disease 162
    Other Causes of Hypertension in Pregnancy 162
    Late or "Transient" Hypertension 163

15 / Optimal Blood Pressure Control 165
    Index 209

CHAPTER 1

INTRODUCTION

THE PREVALENCE OF hypertension in the United States varies with the age, race, and sex of the group under consideration and the definition of hypertension. If a diagnostic cutoff of 140/90 mm Hg or greater is used, more than 60 million Americans are involved.[1] If a diastolic cutoff of 95 mm Hg is used, about 37,330,000 adults are afflicted.[2] The prevalence of hypertension is about twofold greater in blacks than in whites, rises sharply during childbearing years, but is somewhat lower in women than in men until middle age.[3] (Fig 1–1). Given contemporary trends for married couples to delay starting families until both partners are established in their careers, it can be predicted that increasing numbers of older women will present with pregnancy, and, since the prevalence of essential hypertension increases with age, obstetricians, internists, and family practitioners will be faced with the problem inherent in managing a hypertensive pregnancy other than preeclampsia. At present, about one third of the cases of hypertension during pregnancy are due to essential hypertension.[4] Thus, a thorough grasp of the problems associated with hypertension—the regulation of the circulation, possible etiologies and their therapeutic implications, hemodynamics, endocrine and renal changes associated with hypertension in pregnancy, and contemporary pharmacologic and nonpharmacologic management of elevated blood pressure—as well as the effect of pregnancy on these factors, is becoming increasingly important.

No less important is an understanding of the pathophysiology and management of pregnancy-induced hypertension or preeclampsia-eclampsia, a disorder that poses a severe threat to the survival of both mother and infant. The etiologic possibilities in pregnancy-induced hypertension differ from those related to essential hypertension, but must be well understood because of the implications for management, e.g.,

1

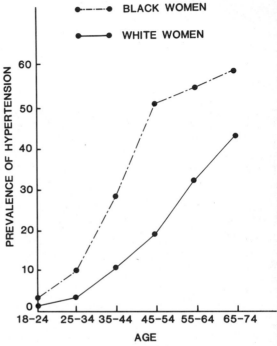

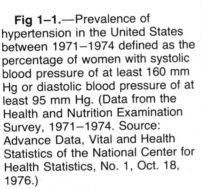

Fig 1–1.—Prevalence of hypertension in the United States between 1971–1974 defined as the percentage of women with systolic blood pressure of at least 160 mm Hg or diastolic blood pressure of at least 95 mm Hg. (Data from the Health and Nutrition Examination Survey, 1971–1974. Source: Advance Data, Vital and Health Statistics of the National Center for Health Statistics, No. 1, Oct. 18, 1976.)

treatment of intravascular coagulation by avoiding interference with prostaglandin synthesis, and preventing unphysiologic contractions of intravascular volume.

To approach the goal of reviewing recent developments in the fields of essential and secondary hypertension accompanying pregnancy and pregnancy-induced hypertension, this monograph will begin with a review of the regulation of the normal circulation and the circulatory adjustments that take place during pregnancy. The various etiologic possibilities in the genesis of essential hypertension and pregnancy-induced hypertension are considered to provide a background for the various management requirements that are discussed later. The consequences of treated and untreated hypertension will be described, to put into perspective the pregnancy that occurs in the long course of essential hypertension and the hypertension that appears only in the relatively brief course of a pregnancy. Finally, the various considerations related to management of the different hypertensive problems associated with pregnancy will be discussed.

CHAPTER 2

CLASSIFICATION

PREGNANCY CAN OCCUR during the long course of chronic hypertension and is sometimes complicated by superimposed preeclampsia. Alternatively, hypertension can be induced by pregnancy in a previously normotensive subject (Fig 2–1). The older term "toxemia of pregnancy" refers to a specific hypertensive disease induced by pregnancy, consisting of two levels of severity, preeclampsia and eclampsia. Preeclampsia is characterized by the appearance of edema, proteinuria, and blood pressure elevation, usually after the 24th week of pregnancy. The term eclampsia refers to the development of seizures and coma. Currently, the phrase "pregnancy-induced hypertension" is used to designate both preeclampsia and eclampsia. Hypertension during pregnancy is a major cause of maternal and perinatal mortality. The incidence of pregnancy-induced hypertension among various groups of primiparas in the United States in recent years ranges from 1.6% to 12.6%. Overall, it is about 7%, increasing to 17% to 86%, depending upon diagnostic criteria, if chronic hypertension predates the pregnancy.[5] However, using an increase of diastolic pressure of 15 mm Hg or more and a sustained urine reaction for protein of 3+ as criteria, Chesley[5] diagnosed superimposed preeclampsia in only 5.7% of gravidas with chronic hypertension. Recurrences occur during approximately 30%, of subsequent pregnancies. The relative frequency of the various forms of hypertension in pregnancy has been examined in several studies. For example, in a London study, 70% of the patients with blood pressure above 120/80 had preeclamptic toxemia, 25% had chronic hypertensive vascular disease, and 5% had chronic nephritis.[6] In a similar series in New York, 72.1% of the patients had specific hypertensive disease of pregnancy, 13.9% had essential hypertension, 5.9% had essential hypertension with superimposed preeclampsia, 1.6% had glomerulonephritis, and 6.3% could not be classified.[7]

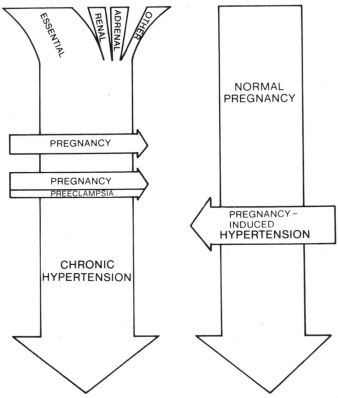

Fig 2–1.—Interrelationships of natural history of hypertension and pregnancy.

One major difficulty in classifying patients lies in making a correct clinical diagnosis. The most certain way appears to be renal biopsy, but this carries a certain degree of risk. The benefit of the information gained must be weighed against a high risk of hemorrhage.[8] In a study of 35 patients with a clinical diagnosis of preeclampsia, characteristic renal pathologic changes were found in only 26%.[9] The severity of glomeruloendotheliosis correlated with serum uric acid but not with blood urea nitrogen (BUN) or serum creatinine, which confirms that a rise in uric acid during pregnancy, in the absence of thiazide administration, provides a way to follow the progression of preeclampsia. In another study, the histologic lesions of chronic renal disease were found in 21% of the multigravidas and 43% of the primagravidas with a clinical diagnosis of preeclampsia, which shows how often these conditions can be confused.[10] Another basis for misdiagnosis lies in the

TABLE 2–1.—A CLASSIFICATION OF ESSENTIAL, SECONDARY AND INDUCED
HYPERTENSION DURING PREGNANCY

I. Preeclampsia-Eclampsia or Pregnancy-Induced
Hypertension
II. Chronic Hypertension
  A. Benign or malignant essential hypertension
    1. Low, normal, or high plasma renin
    2. Normal or high cardiac index
    3. Normal or high plasma norepinephrine
    4. Normal or high plasma volume
  B. Secondary Hypertension
    1. Renal
      a. Renal parenchymal
      b. Renovascular
      c. Renal tumor
    2. Adrenal
      a. Pheochromocytoma
      b. Primary aldosteronism
      c. Cushing's disease
      d. Other forms of mineralocorticoid excess
    3. Miscellaneous
      a. Coarctation or congenital hypoplasia of the aorta
      b. Central nervous system lesions
      c. Other
III. Chronic Hypertension with Superimposed Preeclampsia
IV. Late, Transient Hypertension

fact that peripheral vascular resistance and blood pressure drop in
early pregnancy, rising toward nonpregnant levels in late pregnancy.
Thus, a patient with undetected essential or secondary hypertension
might present in early pregnancy with a blood pressure within normal
limits, only to be misdiagnosed as having preeclampsia when elevated
blood pressure is detected later in the course of pregnancy, especially
if the blood pressure elevation is accompanied by the mild edema that
is frequently seen in otherwise normal pregnancies.

A widely used classification of the hypertensive disorders of pregnancy has been recommended by a committee of the American College
of Obstetricians and Gynecologists. This classification consists of four
groups:

1. Pregnancy induced hypertension, or preeclampsia-eclampsia
2. Chronic hypertension of whatever cause
3. Chronic hypertension with superimposed preeclampsia
4. Late or "transient" hypertension

In the evaluation of individual patients, the physician must expand
group II in order to form a differential diagnosis with different implications for management. This group is first divided into essential hy-

TABLE 2–2.—TYPES OF HYPERTENSION*

I. Systolic and diastolic hypertension
  A. Primary, essential, or idiopathic
  B. Secondary
    1. Renal
      a. Renal parenchymal disease
        (1) Acute glomerulonephritis
        (2) Chronic nephritis
        (3) Polycystic disease
        (4) Connective tissue diseases
        (5) Diabetic nephropathy
        (6) Hydronephrosis
      b. Renovascular
      c. Renin-producing tumors
      d. Renoprival
      e. Primary sodium retention (Liddle's syndrome, Gordon's syndrome)
    2. Endocrine
      a. Acromegaly
      b. Hypothyroidism
      c. Hypercalcemia
      d. Hyperthyroidism
      e. Adrenal
        (1) Cortical
          (a) Cushing's syndrome
          (b) Primary aldosteronism
          (c) Congenital adrenal hyperplasia
        (2) Medullary: pheochromocytoma
      f. Extra-adrenal chromaffin tumor
      g. Carcinoid
      h. Exogenous hormones
        (1) Estrogen
        (2) Glucocorticoids
        (3) Mineralocorticoids: licorice, carbenoxolone
        (4) Sympathomimetics
        (5) Tyramine-containing foods and monoamine oxidase inhibitors
    3. Coarctation of the aorta
    4. Pregnancy-induced hypertension
    5. Neurologic disorders
      a. Increased intracranial pressure
        (1) Brain tumor
        (2) Encephalitis
        (3) Respiratory acidosis: lung or CNS disease
      b. Quadriplegia
      c. Acute porphyria
      d. Familial dysautonomia
      e. Lead poisoning
      f. Guillain-Barré syndrome
    6. Acute stress, including surgery
      a. Psychogenic hyperventilation
      b. Hypoglycemia
      c. Burns
      d. Pancreatitis
      e. Alcohol withdrawal

TABLE 2–2.—Cont'd.

    f. Sickle cell crisis
    g. Postresuscitation
    h. Postoperative
  7. Increased intravascular volume
  8. Drugs and other substances
II. Systolic hypertension
  A. Increased cardiac output
    1. Aortic valvular regurgitation
    2. Arteriovenous fistula, patent ductus
    3. Thyrotoxicosis
    4. Paget's disease of bone
    5. Beriberi
    6. Hyperkinetic circulation
  B. Rigidity of aorta

*From Kaplan N.M.: Systemic hypertension: Mechanisms and diagnosis, in Braunwald E. (ed.): *Heart Disease: A Textbook of Cardiovascular Medicine*, ed. 2. Philadelphia, W.B. Saunders Co., 1984. Used by permission.

pertension and secondary hypertension. Essential hypertension during pregnancy can be of varying degrees of severity and accompanied by varying degrees of damage to target organs, i.e., the central nervous system, retina, heart, and kidneys (Table 2–1). Although Table 2–1 is far from complete, it includes those conditions which have been most often reported to be problems during pregnancy. Table 2–2 contains a more complete list of disorders associated with elevated blood pressure, which includes infrequently encountered diseases. Although rare, many of these conditions can be encountered in pregnant women.

CHAPTER 3

REGULATION OF THE CIRCULATION

THE CIRCULATORY SYSTEM allows absorption of oxygen from the atmosphere and food products from the gut, arranges distribution of these compounds to cells throughout the body, and transports water, carbon dioxide, and other waste products from the cells to lung, kidney, and skin for excretion (Fig 3–1). This function is served by the circulation of blood throughout the body under the driving force of pressure generated by the heart. Thus, in considering the problems of arterial hypertension, one must recall the basic components of the circulatory system: the ventricles, which are pressure generating pumps; the aorta and other large elastic and muscular arteries, which serve as conduits; the resistance arterioles, which allow diffusion of materials into and out of cells; and the venules, veins, and atria, which serve as capacitance vessels, i.e., chambers capable of storing a wide range of blood volumes without major changes in pressure.[11] The circulatory system is capable of intrinsic regulation due to the physical properties of its components and of autoregulation in each of the tissues it serves. The circulatory system is under the overall integrative control of the autonomic nervous system, which regulates function in response to changing physiologic circumstances.

The hemodynamic expression of Ohm's law helps one to understand how the circulation is controlled. Ohm stated that electrical voltage equaled the product of current (amperage) and resistance (ohms). Similarly, the Poiseuille equation for flow of homogeneous fluids states:

$$\text{Flow} = \frac{(\text{pressure gradient}) (\text{vessel radius})^4}{(\text{vessel length}) (\text{viscosity})} \frac{\pi}{8}$$

9

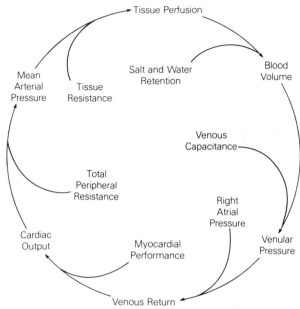

Fig 3–1.—Regulation of the circulation: interplay of factors to maintain arterial pressure and tissue perfusion. (From Sullivan J.M.: Arterial hypertension, in Blacklow R.S. (ed.): *McBryde's Signs and Symptoms*, ed. 6. Philadelphia, J. B. Lippincott, Co., 1983. Used by permission.)

Since vessel length and blood viscosity usually do not vary greatly in a given individual, this equation can be simplified to state:

$$\text{flow} = (\text{pressure})/(\text{resistance})$$

or

$$\text{resistance} = \frac{(\text{arterial pressure})}{(\text{cardiac output})}$$

or

$$\text{arterial pressure} = (\text{cardiac output})(\text{total peripheral resistance})$$

Resistance is a ratio that relates pressure and flow and is an approximation of the vasomotor tone of the vascular smooth muscle fibers in the resistance arterioles. These arterioles are influenced by both remote and local factors.[12] (Fig 3–2). Impulses traveling through the vasoconstrictor fibers of the sympathetic nervous system increase resistance, while fibers in the parasympathetic nervous system have a weak vasodilatory effect. The circulation also carries and delivers to the resistance arterioles vasoactive compounds such as catecholamines, angiotensin II, vasopressin, serotonin, histamine, bradykinin, and certain of the prostaglandins that act directly to alter vasomotor tone.

A number of local factors have important effects on vascular smooth muscle. In metabolically active tissues, the consumption of oxygen and the release of adenosine, hydrogen ions, and potassium ions are associated with vasodilatation as the tissue autoregulates local blood flow. Adenosine is a very powerful vasodilator which is particularly important in the regulation of coronary blood flow. Vascular smooth muscle cells are myogenically active and display slow, rhythmic contraction due to spontaneous depolarization. The stretching effect of arterial blood pressure also stimulates contraction of vascular smooth muscles, an effect originally described by Bayliss.[13] Finally, accumulation of sodium ions in vascular smooth muscle increases sensitivity to circulating angiotensin II and catecholamines[14] and contributes to an elevated vascular resistance.

The second major component in the regulation of blood pressure is cardiac output, the product of heart rate and stroke volume. Heart rate is determined by the intrinsic rate of spontaneous depolarization and repolarization of the sinoatrial node of the heart. Heart rate is regulated by the counterbalancing influences of the stimulatory sympathetic and

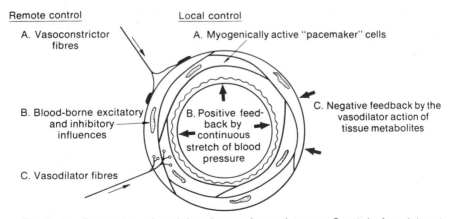

Remote control

A. Vasoconstrictor fibres

B. Blood-borne excitatory and inhibitory influences

C. Vasodilator fibres

Local control

A. Myogenically active "pacemaker" cells

B. Positive feedback by continuous stretch of blood pressure

C. Negative feedback by the vasodilator action of tissue metabolites

Fig 3–2.—Regulation of peripheral vascular resistance. Control of peripheral vascular resistance by local and remote influences, illustrating sites at which prostaglandins and kinins could interact with other control mechanisms to alter vascular tone. (From Folkow B. and Neil E.: *Circulation.* New York, Oxford University Press, 1971. Used by permission.)

inhibitory parasympathetic nervous systems. Blood-borne substances, such as the catecholamines, also influence the heart rate.

The other determinant of cardiac output is stroke volume, which, in turn, is determined by the size of the left ventricle at the end of diastole and the extent of myocardial fiber shortening during systole. Fiber shortening is determined by preload, afterload, and contractility. Preload can be defined as the degree of stretch of the myocardial fibers at the end of diastole. This results from the filling pressure and the compliance characteristics of the ventricle. The filling pressure reflects both venous tone and intravascular volume. As the ventricle increases in size, the amount of blood ejected increases until a plateau is reached, at which point further increases in size fail to increase ventricular performance. Contractility relates ventricular performance to end-diastolic length. When a heart fails, a given fiber length elicits a less than normal contraction; thus contractility is increased when catecholamines stimulate the heart, the same degree of stretch leads to a greater contraction, and contractility is said to be increased. In the intact heart, afterload refers to systolic myocardial wall tension, which is determined by intraventricular pressure and by ventricular size. When preload and contractility are held constant, decreased afterload increases myocardial fiber shortening. A decrease in venous return reduces preload and left ventricular systolic pressure. Thus, afterload can be altered in either of two ways: by reducing arterial pressure or by decreasing ventricular diastolic dimensions.

CHAPTER 4

CIRCULATORY ADJUSTMENTS TO PREGNANCY

FOLLOWING IMPLANTATION OF the fertilized ovum, a series of circulatory adjustments begin that insure an adequate supply of oxygen-rich blood for the developing fetus. These changes involve total blood volume, cardiac output, and total peripheral resistance, among others. Which adjustment occurs first, and to what degree the initial change influences the others, is not yet known. However, it is clear that early in pregnancy, the vascular resistance of uterine blood vessels falls, allowing greater blood flow to the uterus.[15] This effect is attributed to hormonal changes, since experiments have shown that estrogens, which are normally elevated in pregnancy, produce such an effect on uterine perfusion in the nonpregnant animal.[16] Additionally, prolactin, which is also released from the pituitary gland during pregnancy, causes a fall in blood pressure despite an increase in blood volume, which indicates either a fall in resistance or an increase of capacitance.[17]

Although uterine blood flow continues to rise through the 32nd week of gestation, the fall in vascular resistance is not limited to the uterine vessels, since blood flow to the kidneys and to the hands also rises early in pregnancy, falling as term approaches.[18, 19] Blood flow to the legs and arms also increases during the second half of pregnancy.[20] Hepatic and cerebral blood flow has not been found to change during pregnancy.[21, 22]

During the first trimester, blood volume begins to increase, reaching a level about 40% above nonpregnant values at the 30th week of gestation.[23, 24] Thereafter, blood volume remains stable or even decreases

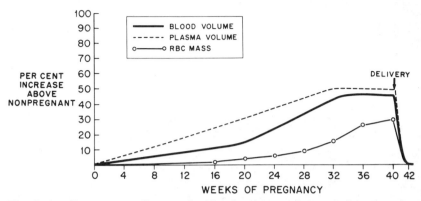

Fig 4–1.—Percentage changes in blood volume, plasma volume, and red blood cell mass during pregnancy. (From Scott D.E.: Anemia in Pregnancy, in Wynn R.M. (ed.): *Obstetrics and Gynecology Annual: 1972*, New York, Appleton-Century-Crofts, 1972. Used by permission.)

slightly, until term (Fig 4–1). Part of the increase in volume results from an increase in the number of erythrocytes, which rise by 20%–40%,[25] but a larger portion of that increase is caused by an expansion of plasma volume, which climbs to a level about 50% greater than nonpregnant values by the 32nd week of pregnancy.[26] The relative difference in red blood cells and plasma volume changes accounts for the "physiologic anemia of pregnancy." The increase in plasma volume is believed to be subsequent to changes in the renin-angiotensin-aldosterone system, which follow the rise in blood progesterone and estrogen levels accompanying a normal pregnancy. Release of renin initiates a sequence that results in salt and water retention, thus expanding plasma volume.[27, 28] The extent to which blood volume increases is proportional to the size of the products of conception, i.e., the blood volume increases more during twin pregnancies than in a single pregnancy.[26] Mean retention of sodium during normal pregnancy has been calculated at 520 mEq, basically the amount required by the conceptus and the increased blood volume.[29] Water is retained in slight excess at term, amounting to 1–2 L in normal pregnancy and 5 L in patients with edema.[30] Edema can occur in a normal pregnancy; Dexter and Weiss originally reported edema in 64% of 100 normal women,[31] and Thompson and co-workers reported edema in 35% of normotensive women during pregnancy.[32] The distribution of this increment in blood volume is not clear. Evidence of increased pulmonary blood volume in early pregnancy has been presented.[33] Routine chest films also suggest an engorgement of the pulmonary vasculature during normal pregnancy. At term, the placental and uterine veins contain large amounts of blood. Uterine blood flow has been measured by the nitrous-oxide method and by uterine-vein cannulation.[34] An average blood flow of 15 ml/100 g/min has been demonstrated in the last month of pregnancy, falling to 9 ml during the first day after delivery. Catheterization of the uterine vein at cesarean section has also shown an average uterine blood flow of 10 ml/100 g/min.[35]

Cardiac output begins to rise during the first 10 weeks of pregnancy,[36] reaching a peak of 30%–45% above resting, nonpregnant levels at around the 20th week (Fig 4–2). Thereafter, the weight of current evidence indicates that cardiac output probably remains elevated until delivery.[37] Pioneer studies in this field were reported by Burwell and co-workers in 1938.[38] Using early gas methods, these investigators made repeated determinations of cardiac output in 4 pregnant patients. They found that cardiac output rose gradually during pregnancy and fell to approach nonpregnant levels during the last months of gestation. This general picture was also found by Hamilton, who measured cardiac output by the Fick method.[39] From the control levels of 4.5 L/

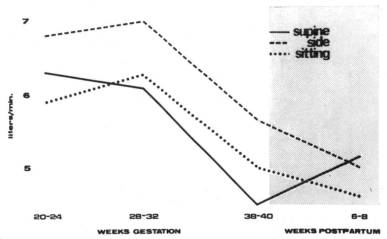

Fig 4–2.—Maternal cardiac output was measured three times during pregnancy and once postpartum in 11 normal women. At each study, measurements were made with the patient sitting, supine, and in left lateral recumbency. Near term, assumption of the supine position causes cardiac output to fall below the postpartum value. (From Ueland K., et al.: Maternal cardiovascular dynamics. IV. The influence of gestational age on the maternal cardiovascular response to posture and exercise. *Am. J. Obstet. Gynecol.* 104:856, 1969. Used by permission.)

min before pregnancy, cardiac output began to rise at the 10th week of gestation, reached a maximum of 5.8 L/min at 26–29 weeks, fell back to 4.6 L/min at 38–40 weeks, then remained at control levels after delivery. However, subsequent investigators have not observed a fall in cardiac output in later pregnancy. This discrepancy is explained by the observation that during pregnancy, cardiac output is very sensitive to changes in position. As the uterus enlarges, it interferes with venous return of blood from the legs by compressing the inferior vena cava, thus reducing cardiac output. This effect is most pronounced in the supine position and is least marked in the left lateral decubitus position.[40, 41, 42] Although an early rise in cardiac output is seen with the patient supine, sitting, or in a lateral decubitis position, cardiac output in the supine patient has been shown to be lower at the end of pregnancy than it is several weeks postpartum.

Heart rate also increases during pregnancy, falling to normal at term. The pulse is faster when the pregnant woman is in the sitting position. Heart rate increases relatively more than cardiac output does in a normal pregnancy, leading to a progressive fall in stroke volume as the pregnancy moves toward term. Stroke volume is lowest in women in late pregnancy who are in the supine position. Stroke volume has been reported to rise to basal levels after delivery.[43]

Even though cardiac output is elevated during pregnancy, the reduced systemic vascular resistance results in either a fall or no change in blood pressure, although the pulse pressure widens. Thus, any elevation of blood pressure before term is a cause for concern. However, a rise in systolic pressure of about 10–15 mm Hg at term is a normal finding (Fig 4–3). The circulatory changes taking place during normal pregnancy resemble those associated with an arteriovenous fistula.[38] Indeed, the oxygen content of mixed venous blood actually rises during normal pregnancy, probably because the rise in oxygen consumption associated with pregnancy is not as great as the rise in cardiac output.[44] Many of these circulatory changes are probably secondary to changes in endocrine function during pregnancy, while others are due to uterine growth and vascular obstruction. In pregnant women, it is characteristic to see a higher resting heart rate, higher cardiac output, higher blood volume, decreased uterine, renal, and peripheral vascular resistance, and increased ventilation.

In addition to the hemodynamic load imposed by the circulatory changes of pregnancy, additional demands are placed on the cardiovascular system during labor and delivery. Because of the added burden, the time around delivery is a time of particular danger for the

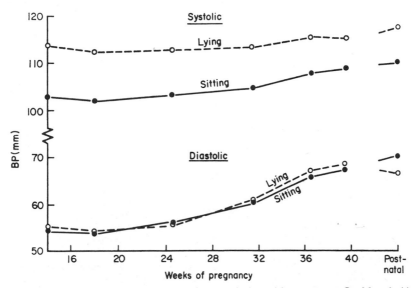

Fig 4–3.—Mean blood pressures of 226 primigravidas seen at St. Mary's Hospital, London. Included are all the patients seen at or before 20 weeks of pregnancy over an 18-month interval. (From MacGillivray I., et al.: Blood pressure survey in pregnancy. *Clin. Sci.* 37:395, 1969. Used by permission.)

woman with cardiovascular disease. Two items are involved: first, the cardiac response to pain accompanying uterine contraction and second, the increased amount of venous blood returning to the heart from the contracting uterus. These factors combine to raise cardiac output by an additional 20% during each uterine contraction.[45]

After delivery, the patient's cardiovascular status gradually returns to normal nonpregnant levels within 1–2 weeks.[46] Additional stresses placed on the circulation at this time result from blood loss during delivery, reabsorption and excretion of the expanded extravascular volume, and the beginning of lactation.

CHAPTER 5

ESSENTIAL HYPERTENSION: ETIOLOGIC CONSIDERATIONS

HEMODYNAMICS OF HUMAN HYPERTENSION

Several studies have shown that patients with mild to moderate essential hypertension have a normal cardiac output.[47] Thus, the increase in blood pressure is accompanied by an increase in total peripheral resistance, the hemodynamic hallmark of established human essential hypertension.

Among patients with the mildest hypertension are those who transiently show elevation of blood pressure to levels above 140/90 mm Hg but who are normal the rest of the time. This has been designated variously "labile" or "borderline" hypertension. Several laboratories have studied the hemodynamic status of this group of hypertensive patients and have found that they differ from those with mild or moderate fixed essential hypertension. The first studies in this area were reported by Widimsky et al.,[48] who studied young patients and found that as a group, these individuals had an elevated cardiac output at rest, a calculated total peripheral resistance that fell within the normal range, and an elevated blood pressure due to the increase in cardiac output. Eich and his co-workers[49] studied an older group of patients with labile hypertension and also found an elevated cardiac output with vascular resistance within the normal range. Several other laboratories have confirmed the finding of an elevated cardiac output in patients of similar description and have also noted that such individuals tend to have a higher left ventricular systolic ejection rate and a faster heart rate, leading several to propose that a disorder of the autonomic nervous system might be involved in the pathogenesis of labile or borderline hypertension. Julius and his coworkers[50] have found a spectrum of hemodynamic changes in individuals with labile hypertension; there are those with a very high cardiac output and those whose cardiac output was relatively reduced. It has been proposed that labile or borderline hypertension is the initial phase of a disease process that eventually leads to sustained elevation of blood pressure and vascular resistance.

A number of studies have been carried out to find a reason for the elevation of cardiac output. Ulrych et al.[51] found that individuals with labile hypertension did not have an increase in intravascular volume. However, intravascular volume appeared to be redistributed towards the central circulation. Thus, an increased amount of blood was present in the cardiopulmonary circulation, increasing venous return to the heart and stimulating an increase in cardiac output via the Starling mechanism.

Another explanation for the increased cardiac output could be increased activity of the autonomic nervous system. The evidence in favor of this hypothesis is that such individuals have an increased heart rate and an increased rate of left ventricular ejection. Julius et al.[52] studied the effect of β-adrenergic blockade and parasympathetic inhibition in young patients with hypertension secondary to an elevated cardiac output and found that this dual blockade resulted in a return of cardiac output to normal levels. They also studied the effect of interventions such as sitting, mild exercise, and infusion of dextran upon the hemodynamics of individuals with borderline hypertension and found that peripheral vascular resistance during any intervention was higher in the labile hypertensives than in the normotensive individuals. Similarly, Sannerstedt and his co-workers[53] have studied the degree to which cardiac output and vascular resistance change with exercise in patients with labile hypertension in comparison with normal patients and have found that the slope of the line relating output to resistance was shifted, indicating that peripheral vascular resistance was actually inappropriately elevated in individuals with mild labile hypertension.

Takeshita and Mark[54] studied the effect of stimuli causing maximum reactive hyperemia on forearm blood flow and resistance in normal subjects and in subjects with borderline hypertension and have demonstrated that forearm vascular resistance fails to fall as greatly during maximum reactive hyperemia in labile hypertensive subjects. It has also been observed that such patients have altered diastolic properties of the left ventricle[55] and attenuation of the microvasculature.[56]

Thus, patients with labile, borderline hypertension are characterized by an increased cardiac output, a central redistribution of blood volume, and evidence of enhanced activity of the autonomic nervous system, leading to an increased heart rate, an increase in left ventricular ejection rate and an inability to decrease forearm vascular resistance adequately in response to circumstances that demand an increase in blood flow.

Essential hypertension can be further subdivided into categories of mild, moderate, and severe, depending upon the degree of elevation of diastolic pressure and the extent of involvement of target organs—the brain, the heart, the kidneys, and the peripheral vasculature. The hemodynamic pattern found in each of these subdivisions of patients appears to be determined by the interplay of three factors. The first relates to the degree of increase of peripheral vascular resistance and blood pressure. The second involves the degree of cardiac hypertrophy compensating for the elevated blood pressure and, later, the degree of impairment of cardiac function. The third factor relates to the extent to which pressure diuresis has taken place, resulting in a gradual contraction of intravascular volume and a redistribution of fluid volumes.

Meerson[57] postulated that ventricular function undergoes three stages of change during the development of hypertension. As afterload increases gradually, a stage of enhanced function of the ventricle occurs due to hypertrophy, during which time the ventricle can perform increased work. During this phase, the heart has been affected by the increased blood pressure, but it can still function normally. Later, hypertrophy no longer suffices to compensate for the increased afterload, and the function of the left ventricle becomes impaired. Initially, this impaired function is subtle and requires very sensitive techniques to detect. Later, the function worsens to the degree that failure is clinically evident. With regard to hypertension during pregnancy, it is important to note that sudden, severe elevation of blood pressure, which does not allow time for compensatory hypertrophy to develop, can lead rapidly to the onset of heart failure.

Early in the natural history of hypertension there is no evidence of cardiac involvement detected by electrocardiogram (ECG) or chest x-ray study. Hemodynamic studies have shown that cardiac output remains normal. However, since vascular resistance and arterial pressure are higher, the ventricular workload is increased. Heart rate tends to be increased, while stroke volume and left ventricular ejection rate, a reflection of ventricular contractility, are normal.

If the hypertensive process continues without treatment, the first evidence of cardiac involvement emerges, with the appearance of a fourth heart sound on physical examination. The ECG may reveal evidence of left atrial enlargement. Measurement of systolic time intervals shows that the preejection period is prolonged at this stage. Heart rate remains elevated and cardiac output remains normal, although ventricular ejection rate begins to fall. At this point, even though the chest x-ray film might not reveal cardiac enlargement, echocardiographic techniques can demonstrate increased thickness of the left ventricular wall.

The progression of the hypertensive process leads to the development of cardiac enlargement that can be seen on chest x-ray film and the appearance of voltage and other criteria for left ventricular hypertrophy on the ECG. At this point, hemodynamic studies reveal further increases in total peripheral resistance and arterial pressure, cardiac output is reduced, even at rest, and systolic ejection rate falls further.

A third factor which has profound influence upon the hemodynamics of severe hypertension is the redistribution of fluid volumes. In human hypertension, studies have not revealed a change in either total body water or in intracellular fluid volume. Thus, attention has focused on the distribution of extracellular fluid.

Over the years, a number of physiologic studies have pointed out that the kidney will increase its output of urine as arterial pressure rises, thus reducing intravascular volume and lowering arterial pressure to the prior level.[58] Guyton and his colleagues[59] have proposed that an impairment of the kidney's ability to respond appropriately to pressure is a major factor in the genesis of essential hypertension (Fig 5–1). It is postulated that the kidney is set to begin pressure diuresis at a higher level in the hypertensive patient. Thus, an individual with an expanded intravascular volume, e.g., secondary to a high-sodium diet, would initially increase cardiac output, thus stimulating autoregulation in individual organs throughout the body, leading to an increase in local, then total, peripheral resistance, an increase in blood pressure, and an increase in urinary excretion of sodium and water, thus restoring cardiac output and intravascular volume to normal at the price of a higher vascular resistance and arterial blood pressure.

Changes in pressure within the blood vessels also serve to redistribute intravascular volume. An increase in intravascular pressure tends

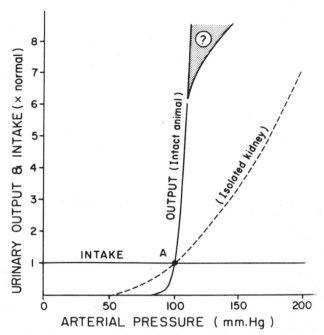

Fig 5–1.—Graphic procedure for analyzing the long-term level of arterial pressure, based on the renal-body fluid mechanism for pressure control. The steep *solid curve* is the normal urinary output curve in an intact animal. (From Guyton A.C.: Regulation of arterial pressure: II. The renal-body fluid system for long-term pressure control. Mechanisms of hypertension, in Guyton A.C.: *Textbook of Medical Physiology*, ed. 5. Philadelphia, W. B. Saunders Co., 1976. Used by permission.)

to increase the transport of water across capillary walls into the interstitial fluid, thus reducing intravascular volume. Similarly, a reduction of pressure is associated with an expansion of intravascular volume as fluid returns from the interstitial spaces. Measurement of interstitial fluid volume in patients with essential hypertension has usually shown that the ratio of plasma volume to interstitial fluid volume is reduced, suggesting that fluid passes through the capillaries into the interstitial spaces due to the high intravascular pressure.

Tarazi[60] studied fluid compartments in several forms of clinical hypertension and demonstrated that as blood pressure rises in the presence of normal renal function, intravascular volume falls on the basis of a decrease in plasma volume (Fig 5–2). The higher the pressure, the lower the intravascular volume, unless significant parenchymal renal disease is present, in which case the level of blood pressure elevation is directly proportional to the plasma volume (Fig 5–3). Thus, individuals with severe hypertension presenting for urgent treatment, such as those with severe preeclampsia, might be expected to have a significantly contracted intravascular volume if they are free of renal failure. Therefore, excessive use of diuretic therapy in such individuals is inappropriate. Similarly, antihypertensive therapy based on the use of vasodilating agents can be expected to decrease intravascular pressure, allowing the return of fluid from the interstitium into the vascular tree, expanding plasma volume, and blunting the antihypertensive effect or pseudotolerance. Thus, careful use of diuretic agents is appropriate to

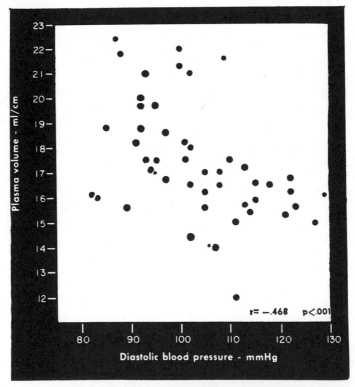

Fig 5–2.—A highly significant inverse relationship between plasma volume and diastolic arterial pressure (average for week) in 47 men with essential hypertension. (From Tarazi R.C., et al.: Plasma volume and chronic hypertension. Relationship to arterial pressure levels in different hypertensive diseases. *Arch. Intern. Med.* 125:835, 1970. Used by permission; copyright 1970, American Medical Association.)

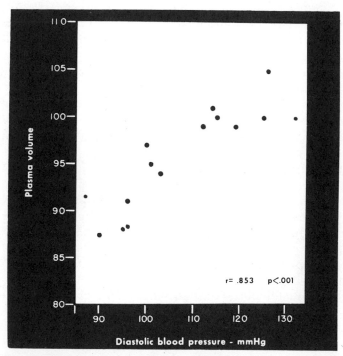

Fig 5–3.—A direct relationship between plasma volume (expressed in percent of normal volume to allow comparison of values for men and women) and diastolic pressure in 16 patients with hypertension accompanying renal parenchymal disease. (From Tarazi R.C., et al.: Plasma volume and chronic hypertension. Relationship to arterial pressure levels in different hypertensive diseases. *Arch. Intern. Med.* 125:835, 1970. Used by permission; copyright 1970, American Medical Association.)

counter this effect when the response to antihypertensive therapy is inadequate.

Increasing degrees of severity of essential hypertension are marked by increases in peripheral vascular resistance. The phase of increased cardiac output, which is characteristic of young labile borderline hypertensives patients, may sometimes persist into the phase of fixed mild essential hypertension and, less frequently, is found in the severely hypertensive patient.[61] Alternatively, cardiac output may be normal in the mildly hypertensive patient. Such individuals do not have clinically measureable damage of heart, kidneys, or brain. At times, patients in this group are found to have redistribution of blood volume to the cardiopulmonary circulation, as is found in a normal pregnant woman.

Such hypertensive subjects also have an increased heart rate and evidence of increased myocardial contractility with a normal stroke volume. The fact that the baroreceptor reflex does not act to slow the heart rate in an attempt to lower blood pressure at this point indicates that the baroreceptors have been reset. Intravascular volume may be mildly reduced in patients of this description.

In patients with moderate essential hypertension, evidence of cardiac involvement can be detected. Careful renal function studies sometimes reveal evidence of early impairment. Total peripheral resistance and arterial blood pressure are higher, cardiac output is ordinarily normal, and heart rate remains greater than normal. In the absence of significant renal damage, plasma volume contracts in proportion to the increase in diastolic blood pressure. As diastolic pressure exceeds 105 mm Hg, the decrease in intravascular volume becomes more apparent. The stroke volume remains normal or may, at this point, start to fall. Myocardial contractility is within the normal range. In this phase, echocardiographic studies may reveal increased thickness of the left ventricular wall.

Severe essential hypertension develops as the diastolic pressure rises

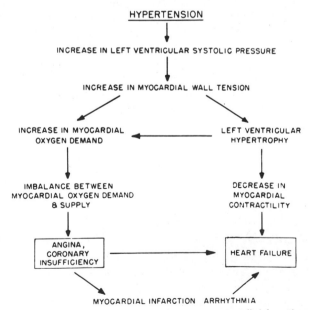

Fig 5–4.—Adverse effects of hypertension on myocardial function. (From Hollander W.: Role of hypertension in atherosclerosis and cardiovascular disease. *Am. J. Cardiol.* 38:786, 1976. Used by permission.)

still further and evidence of target-organ damage emerges clinically. The chest x-ray film and ECG begin to reveal evidence of cardiac enlargement and hypertrophy. Renal function studies reveal the first evidence of a decrease in creatinine clearance and perhaps a minor increase in BUN. The hemodynamic characteristic of this phase of hypertension is an even higher total peripheral resistance. Although left ventricular hypertrophy is present, cardiac output may begin to fall. Heart rate might remain elevated but stroke volume is lower. Plasma volume decreases still further, and, as cardiac output and intravascular volume fall, plasma renin activity usually rises. Since arterial blood pressure is severely increased in this phase and cardiac enlargement has occurred, the left ventricular tension generated during each contraction is greatly increased, making contraction increasingly difficult, and leading, if not treated, to the development of pulmonary edema (Fig 5–4).

SODIUM, THE KIDNEY, AND THE HEART

The cardiovascular system is influenced by sodium. Dietary intake of sodium has been proposed to be an important influence in the development of high blood pressure.[62] If untreated, high blood pressure affects the heart by predisposing to the development of left ventricular hypertrophy, congestive heart failure, coronary artery disease, and other cardiovascular disorders. The prevalence of hypertension has been shown to vary directly with sodium intake in a number of populations. However, even in populations that consume enormous quantities of sodium, e.g., the northern Japanese, who ingest 25 g of salt daily, the majority of individuals do not become hypertensive; only 35%–40% develop hypertension in northern Japan.[63] It has been shown that stringent sodium restriction sometimes reduces blood pressure[64] and extracellular fluid.[65] It has also been observed that moderate salt restriction lowers average blood pressure by about 8/4 mm Hg.[66] However, all individuals do not respond to sodium restriction with a fall in blood pressure.[67] These observations suggest that certain individuals are more sensitive to sodium than others. At present, we lack the clinical means to identify reliably the sodium-sensitive individual.

The mechanism by which sodium chloride ingestion results in blood pressure elevation has not been clearly defined. One proposal, derived

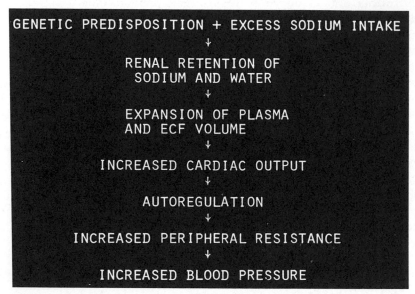

Fig 5–5.—Possible sequence of events leading to the development of chronic essential hypertension in sodium-sensitive individuals.

from a number of lines of experimental evidence, suggests that excessive intake of sodium chloride leads to sodium and water retention, expansion of extracellular fluid and intravascular volume, increased venous return, and elevated cardiac index. As elevated blood flow to the tissues continues, whole-body autoregulation takes place, with a subsequent increase in total peripheral resistance and the eventual development of hypertension.[58] The elevated blood pressure leads to increased urine output and restoration of extracellular fluid and cardiac index to normal, while hypertension is sustained because of the elevated vascular resistance (Fig 5–5). Guyton and his co-workers have used systems analysis to study the problem and have derived data which support this general outline.[59] In studies of the relative effects of the various feedback loops involved in blood pressure control, they have concluded that chronic blood pressure elevation will not occur unless the kidney fails to increase salt and water excretion appropriately and therefore does not reduce extracellular fluid and arterial blood pressure back to normal.

Certain animal experiments have supported this proposal. Coleman and Guyton have shown that the loading of sodium and water in dogs with reduced renal mass causes a chronic expansion of extracellular

fluid, followed by a series of events similar to those observed by Ledingham in rats with renovascular hypertension: sequential elevation of
cardiac index, vascular resistance, and blood pressure, and increased
urine output, ultimately lowered extracellular fluid.[68] Dahl[69] has selec-
tively inbred strains of rats to produce groups that invariably develop
hypertension when fed salt and other groups that are resistant to hypertension despite sodium loading, a circumstance similar to the human experience. Bianchi[70] and Dahl[71] have transplanted the kidneys of
sodium-resistant rats into hypertensive sodium-sensitive rats, who
subsequently became normotensive. Transplantation of kidneys from
hypertensive rats has succeeded in making sodium-resistant rats sodium-sensitive, which suggests that the genetic predisposition to sodium sensitivity resides in the kidney. In parabiotic experiments,
Dahl[72] and his co-workers have demonstrated transmittal from the
plasma of sodium-sensitive animals a humeral factor that raises the
blood pressure of sodium-resistant rats. Tobian et al. have produced
chronic hypertension in rats fed 8% sodium for 4 months[73] and have
observed that the kidneys of sodium-sensitive rats require a higher
level of perfusion pressure for a given amount of sodium excretion.
Ganguli et al.[74] have studied the hemodynamic effects of sodium loading in Dahl "S" (sensitive) and "R" (resistant) rats and observed that
the sodium-resistant rats responded with vasodilation that allowed
blood pressure to remain normal despite an increased cardiac index. In
contrast, the sodium-sensitive rats responded with an increase in blood
pressure, cardiac index, and vascular resistance. Vascular resistance increased with time as the cardiac index fell to control levels. The elevated blood pressure was maintained by the increased vascular resistance.

Cardiac function and sodium homeostasis are interrelated in a number of fascinating ways that might influence the way that an individual
responds to sodium. One of the most interesting recent findings in this
area has been the discovery of atrial natriuretic factor. Granular structures in the atria, interposed among myocytes, were described by
Kisch[75] in 1956. DeBold[76] later observed that these granules were altered by changes in water and electrolyte balance and, with his co-
workers, reported that atrial extracts caused a rapid and potent natriuretic response.[77] Subsequent studies have shown that atrial natriuretic
factor has a molecular weight of 5,000 to 30,000 daltons, contains one
or more peptide fragments, relaxes vascular and intestinal smooth
muscle, lowers blood pressure, and does not inhibit sodium-potassium
adenosine triphosphatase (ATPase) or change glomerular filtration

rate. Natriuresis takes place because atrial natriuretic factor inhibits re-sorption of sodium, potassium, chloride, and water in the renal tubule, probably distal to the loop of Henle.[78] A deficiency of this factor could underlie sodium sensitivity.

In addition to their hormonal function, the left atrium and posterior left ventricle also contain stretch receptors[79] that respond to sodium-induced changes in heart size. As left atrial size increases, the receptors are activated, vagal afferent nerve traffic increases, and heart rate, total peripheral resistance, and blood pressure fall. Further, the release of antidiuretic hormone (ADH) is inhibited and water excretion increases, thus reducing heart size. Renal blood flow, glomerular filtration rate, and sodium excretion increase, since stimulation of the stretch recep-tors also decreases efferent nerve traffic to the kidney, which in turn reduces renin release, angiotensin II formation, and aldosterone secre-tion. With chronic increases in heart size, the sensitivity of atrial and ventricular receptors decreases, thereby reducing the capacity to re-store fluid components to normal levels. Impaired receptor function could explain why vascular resistance does not fall appropriately in sodium-sensitive individuals when heart size is increased by a high sodium intake.

Expansion of intravascular volume by sodium-loading in volume-dependent forms of experimental hypertension leads to the appearance in plasma of a digoxin-like substance, endoxin.[80] This nonpeptide com-pound, of less than 500-dalton molecular weight, inhibits sodium-po-tassium ATPase, thus preventing resorption of sodium throughout the renal tubule and causing natriuresis. However, by inhibiting sodium-potassium ATPase throughout the body, particularly in vascular smooth muscle, endoxin leads to intracellular accumulation of sodium, then of calcium, thus causing vasoconstriction and elevation of blood pressure.[81] Hamlyn et al.[82] have observed that plasma levels of a so-dium-potassium ATPase inhibitor are proportional to the level of blood pressure in patients with essential hypertension. Such a substance could have an important influence on the way an individual responds to dietary sodium.

In studies of normotensive volunteers, Kirkendall et al. have found that a 400-mEq sodium diet increased forearm blood flow without an increase in blood pressure or in right atrial pressure, thus suggesting that local vasodilatation took place.[83] Mark et al.[84] found that patients with borderline hypertension had decreased forearm blood flow when they were salt loaded, suggesting that sodium acts to cause vasocon-striction in such patients. Studies of patients with labile[85] or mild es-

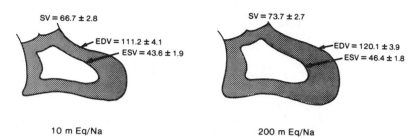

SV = 66.7 ± 2.8

EDV = 111.2 ± 4.1
ESV = 43.6 ± 1.9

SV = 73.7 ± 2.7

EDV = 120.1 ± 3.9
ESV = 46.4 ± 1.8

10 m Eq/Na   200 m Eq/Na

Fig 5–6.—Effect of sodium intake on heart size and stroke volume. (From Sullivan J.M.: Sodium and the heart, in Messerli F.H. (ed.): *The Heart in Hypertension.* New York, Yorke Medical Books, 1985. Used by permission.)

sential hypertension[86] have shown normal extracellular fluid and/or plasma volumes but have demonstrated elevated cardiac index and normal vascular resistance. These studies suggest that these patients are in but one phase of hypertension development and will later develop elevated vascular resistance if their tissues undergo autoregulation. Whether sodium intake contributes to this elevation of cardiac index in man is not known.

Sullivan et al.,[87] using echocardiographic techniques to study each subject as their own control, have made serial measurements of cardiac index during states of high- and low-sodium intake. First, they observed that a high-sodium diet increased heart size and stroke volume[87] (Fig 5–6). They subsequently found that a 200-mEq sodium diet, given after a period of sodium restriction, results in a 5% or greater increase in mean blood pressure in about 40% of borderline hypertensive subjects but in only 22% of normal subjects.[88] The normal subjects responded to sodium repletion with an increase in cardiac index and a fall in total peripheral resistance. The response in the hypertensive subjects was more varied: of those showing an increase in blood pressure, 50% did so because of an increase in cardiac index without an adequate fall in vascular resistance, and the other 50% because of a rise in vascular resistance, which suggests that the human population of North America is far less genetically homogenous than the Dahl sodium-sensitive rat. Whether these changes persist, and which, if any, are associated with the eventual development of hypertension are important unanswered questions. Sullivan and Ratts[89] have found that the increased cardiac index and decreased vascular resistance persist during 12 months of liberal sodium intake in sodium-resistant subjects; these are hemodynamic changes resembling those of a normal pregnancy (Fig 5–7). Sullivan and Ratts have found also that

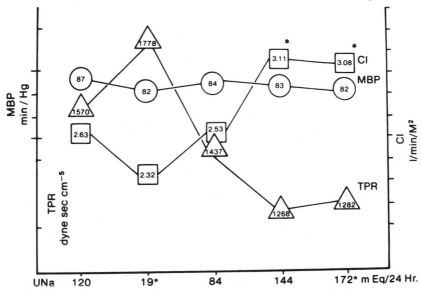

Fig 5–7.—Adaptation to daily sodium intake of approximately 200 mEq by 10 normotensive sodium resistant subjects. The first three observations were 5 days apart, while the fourth period (144 mEq sodium excretion) was 6 months later, and the fifth period (172 mEq sodium) was 1 year later. (Adapted from Sullivan J.M., Ratts T.R.: Hemodynamic mechanisms of adaptation to chronic high sodium intake in normal humans. *Hypertension* 5:814, 1983.)

blood pressure remained elevated at 6 months in sodium-sensitive subjects because of an inadequate fall in resistance.

This heterogeneity of response has been found by other investigators under different circumstances. In patients requiring chronic hemodialysis, Onesti et al.[90] found that expansion of extracellular fluid between dialysis did not cause an increase in vascular resistance or blood pressure in previously normotensive subjects, while blood pressure rose along with resistance in 60%, or with cardiac index in 20%, of the hypertensive patients. Similarly, Bravo et al.[91] have found that mineralocorticoid-induced hypertension in the dog was, in some cases, associated with an increased resistance and in other cases with an increased cardiac index. Berecek and Bohr[92] have made similar observations in the pig. Luft et al.[93] have studied the hemodynamic and metabolic response of normal subjects to extremes of sodium intake, 10 to 1,500 mEq daily. They found that an intake of 800 mEq or more was associated with a significant increase in average blood pressure and in cardiac index.

Epidemiologic studies also suggest a link between potassium deficiency and hypertension.[94] Direct infusion of potassium chloride and slight increases in serum potassium concentration have been found to have a vasodilatory effect in several vascular beds in man and in experimental animals.[95, 96] Evidence has been presented to suggest that this vasodilator effect is attenuated in hypertensive humans.[97] Potassium has natriuretic effects, due to decreased tubular absorption of sodium. Luft et al.[98] have found that potassium replacement promotes saluresis and reduces the blood pressure-elevating effects of sodium in normal subjects. MacGregor et al.[99] found that potassium supplementation lowered blood pressure in hypertensive subjects. Thus, potassium might be an important modifier of the effects of sodium on the cardiovascular system.

Impaired left ventricular diastolic function has been found in patients with cardiac hypertrophy.[100] Al Aouar et al. observed that the maximum left ventricular filling rates in young, borderline hypertensive patients without left ventricular hypertrophy[55] did not vary as heart size was altered by variations in sodium intake as did the filling rates in normal subjects. Recently, Ratts et al.[101] reported that of a group of patients presenting with chronic hypertension and heart failure of recent onset, only 39% had echocardiographic evidence of impaired left ventricular contraction, and of these, 91% had a history of alcoholism, prior myocardial infarction, or other illness that could explain abnormal left ventricular function. Fully 61% had normal systolic shortening despite hypertrophied ventricles, suggesting that sodium-induced volume overload, plus a stiff left ventricle with abnormal diastolic relaxation, explained the development of pulmonary congestion.

Thus, in normal, sodium-resistant individuals, a high-sodium diet results in an increase in left ventricular end-diastolic and end-systolic size, and an increase in stroke volume and in cardiac index. These changes are accommodated by a fall in total peripheral resistance, which in turn maintains arterial blood pressure at usual levels. The sodium-sensitive individual usually shows the same cardiac response, but his vascular resistance does not lower to the same degree or may even vasoconstrict, therefore blood pressure rises. The reason for this abnormal interplay between flow and resistance remains to be discovered.

These observations suggest that perhaps as many as 40% of women with chronic essential hypertension could be sodium-sensitive, and that the efforts to correct the contraction of plasma volume, which can be expected to accompany chronic hypertension, might result in further elevation of blood pressure. In addition, the stiff left ventricle with impaired diastolic function that is found in otherwise healthy individuals with chronic hypertension could result in a marked rise in left ventricular filling pressure and pulmonary capillary pressure if such individuals receive a sudden saline load, such as an aggressive attempt to correct intravascular volume contraction with saline administered intravenously in a patient with hypertension during pregnancy, without appropriate invasive hemodynamic monitoring.

ACTIVITY OF THE SYMPATHETIC NERVOUS SYSTEM

A large number of inconclusive reports published over several years continue to prompt investigation of a possible role for the sympathetic nervous system in either initiating or sustaining essential hypertension. Several lines of evidence contribute to this sustained interest. The first is that patients with pheochromocytoma and high serum levels of epinephrine/norepinephrine have high blood pressure that usually returns to normal when the tumor is removed and catecholamine levels return to normal. Second, patients with essential hypertension have higher resting pulse rates than patients with normal blood pressure.[85] Third, patients with essential hypertension respond favorably to therapy with agents that interfere with the action of the sympathetic nervous system at several different levels. Fourth, recent studies have found elevated levels of norepinephrine in the plasma of certain patients with essential hypertension, but the overlap with normotensive patients was quite extensive.[102, 103, 104] Fifth, plasma levels of dopamine-β-hydroxylase, which are believed to reflect the activity of peripheral sympathetic nerve endings, correlate closely with diastolic blood pressure levels in hypertensive subjects.[105, 106]

Part of the difficulty in establishing a role for the sympathetic nervous system, or in eliminating this possibility, has been methodologic. Early studies relied on relatively insensitive bioassay or spectrophotofluorometric techniques. More recent studies carried out with the more sensitive double isotope technique have supported a role for the sympathetic nervous system, although this point has not been established conclusively.[107] Lewis, Doyle, and Anavekar[106] have studied plasma norepinephrine levels in 31 patients with essential hypertension and found a significant individual correlation between plasma norepinephrine concentration and simultaneous arterial pressure. They also found an impressive correlation between plasma norepinephrine levels and the effects of treatment with ganglionic blocking agents on systolic atrial pressure. These are the most convincing correlations available, but they still do not prove the point that the sympathetic nervous system is more active in those patients with essential hypertension than in normal subjects.

It has been assumed that the excretion of the metabolic breakdown products of epinephrine and norepinephrine is a reflection of endogenous sympathetic nervous system activity, even though the levels of these products do not reflect the amount of norepinephrine that undergoes reuptake by the nerve endings after stimulus and release. In support of this postulate is the observation that urinary excretion of metabolites increases with upright posture or after sympathetic or ganglionic blockade. A recent review of studies in which these compounds have been measured in patients with essential hypertension shows conflicting results.[108] Vanillylmandelic acid excretion has been found to be elevated in one study, unchanged in two others, and down in a fourth study. Total metanephrine excretion has also been inconsistent, with two studies reporting normal levels and two groups observing an elevation. Likewise, norepinephrine excretion has been found to be normal in ten studies, up in two, and down in one, while dopamine excretion has been found to be normal in two studies and decreased in one. Gitlow and his co-workers found elevated plasma norepinephrine clearance rates in patients with essential hypertension, but DeQuattro and Sjoerdsma usually found normal rates except for patients who also had elevated urinary norepinephrine levels.[109, 110]

Several questions regarding the sympathetic nervous system in patients with essential hypertension remain to be answered, i.e., why do some patients with serum norepinephrine levels equivalent to those of patients with essential hypertension have normal blood pressures? Would correction of elevated norepinephrine levels invariably restore normal blood pressure? Are there differences in levels among patients with early labile hypertension, patients with fixed essential hypertension of long duration, and those with severe or malignant hypertension? Is there a relationship between circulating levels of norepinephrine and activity of the renin-angiotensin system, and does this relationship differ between normotensive and hypertensive subjects?

At centers in which accurate measurement of plasma norepinephrine levels can be obtained and the normal range can be well established, therapy for the nonpregnant patient who is found to have elevated levels can be planned to take advantage of the effects of the centrally acting α receptor agonists or agents that block the sympathetic nervous system peripherally. In theory, β-adrenergic receptor blockers should not be very effective in this group, because the α-adrenergic receptors would not be blocked and would respond to elevated norepinephrine levels by increasing peripheral vascular resistance. However, if the elevated blood pressure is due to an elevated cardiac output, blockade of β_1 receptions should lower pressure.

In clinics that do not have access to plasma norepinephrine determinations, a clue to the presence of elevated activity of the sympathetic nervous system can be provided by a rapid heart rate, a hyperdynamic precordium, or the finding of orthostatic hypertension. When mean arterial blood pressure climbs by 10 mm Hg or more when the patient assumes an upright position, orthostatic hypertension is present and suggests overactivity of the sympathetic nervous system.

The pregnant patient with chronic hypertension responds well to reduction of sympathetic activity with methyldopa, but she also responds to antihypertensive measures that do not involve the sympathetic nervous system directly. At present, there is no compelling clinical reason to measure plasma catecholamine levels to guide therapy during pregnancy, other than to exclude pheochromocytoma.

THE RENIN-ANGIOTENSIN-ALDOSTERONE SYSTEM

The known association between nephritis and hypertension led Tigerstedt and Bergman to seek pressor substances in the kidney.[111] In 1898, they published studies on the hemodynamic effects of crude saline extracts of rabbit kidney. The saline extracts caused a rise in blood pressure within 10 seconds, peaking at 2 minutes, and disappearing by 20 minutes. In 1934, Goldblatt produced hypertension by partial occlusion of the renal artery of the dog.[112] In 1939, Page observed that renin, mixed with saline and injected into an ear vessel, did not cause vasoconstriction, but was a vasoconstrictor when mixed with blood,[113] suggesting that renin must interact with blood before a pressor substance was formed. Also in 1939, Braun-Meńendez found a pressor substance in renal vein blood, which did not have the physical properties of renin and eventually proved to be angiotensin.[114] In 1953, Simpson and his co-workers purified aldosterone.[115] In 1955, as a result of work from a number of laboratories, angiotensin I and II were isolated and the angiotensin-converting enzyme was described. In 1960, Laragh et al.[116] and Genest and his co-workers[117] found elevated aldosterone excretion in patients with malignant hypertension and, in 1960, Laragh observed that infusion of angiotensin II caused increased urinary aldosterone excretion. Thus, the components forming a feedback loop were uncovered (Fig 5–8). The liver synthesizes renin substrate, a glycoprotein that is released into the circulation. Renin, a proteolytic enzyme, cleaves a decapeptide, angiotensin I, from the substrate molecule. During passage through the pulmonary circulation, angiotensin I is lysed by converting enzyme, leaving the octapeptide angiotensin II, a potent vasopressor, which is eventually destroyed by angiotensinases. Angiotensin II has several effects, among which are vasoconstriction, facilitation of norepinephrine release, and aldosterone release, which in turn causes sodium retention in the distal tubules of the kidney. Evidence exists that the aldosterone effect might be mediated by a heptapeptide, angiotensin III.[118]

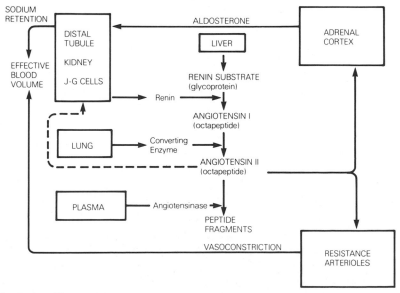

Fig 5–8.—The renin-angiotensin-aldosterone feedback loop for the regulation of effective blood volume. (From Sullivan J.M.: Arterial hypertension, in Blacklow R.S. (ed.): *McBryde's Signs and Symptoms*, ed. 6. Philadelphia, J. B. Lippincott, Co., 1983. Used by permission.)

The renin-angiotensin system acts to maintain blood pressure in two major ways by increasing effective blood volume and by increasing peripheral vascular resistance. In addition, angiotensin II acts directly on the juxtaglomerular cells to inhibit renin release, thus acting as a brake on the system. Any manipulation that tends to reduce blood pressure, blood volume, or sodium concentration tends to activate the feedback loop. Pregnancy, hemorrhage, hypotension, sodium depletion, gastrointestinal fluid loss, upright posture, and renal artery stenosis all stimulate renin release.

The control of renin release is complicated and involves the interplay of a number of factors as the body adjusts to changing circumstances. The major factors involved are: the vascular receptor in the afferent renal arteriole, the macula densa, the sympathetic nervous system, and several blood-borne substances.[119] The vascular receptor is comprised of the juxtaglomerular cells and portions of the afferent glomerular arteriole. This receptor responds to changes in wall tension caused by changes in perfusion pressure,[120] sympathetic nerve activity,[121] and intrinsic changes in vascular smooth muscle during renal autoregulation.[122] The macula densa reponds to changes in the rate of sodium delivery,[123] but the relative importance of this mechanism in the control of renin release is not clear. A number of agents are known to effect renin release, including sodium,[124] potassium,[125] angiotensin II,[126] catecholamines,[127] estrogens,[128] adrenal steroids,[129] ADH,[130] and prostaglandins.[131, 132]

Although the renal sympathetic nerves are an important modulating factor in the control of renin release, they are not essential. Increased renin secretion in response to sodium depletion has been demonstrated in dogs with bilateral renal denervation.[133] In experimental animals, it has been shown that β-adrenergic receptor blockade prevents the increase in renin secretion produced by hypoglycemia,[134] brain stem stimulation,[135] infusion of catecholamines,[136] acute hemorrhage, adrenalectomy, chronic salt depletion, and acute renal artery constriction.[137] Although evidence has been presented to show that renin secretion is also prevented by α-adrenergic receptor blockade,[136] other laboratories have observed that agents which block α-adrenergic receptors actually potentiate stimulated renin release.[138, 139] Human studies have shown that small, intravenously administered doses of propranolol promptly suppress renin release,[140] while studies of longer duration have yielded variable results. Propranolol, taken orally, has been reported to lower blood pressure and plasma renin activity proportionately,[141] to lower renin activity without affecting blood pressure in patients with renovascular hypertension,[142] to block the rise in plasma renin activity that follows diuretic therapy or upright posture,[143] and to lower blood pressure without affecting renin activity in patients receiving diuretics.[144] An exaggerated plasma renin response to salt depletion has been observed in patients on long-term propranolol therapy.[145]

Aldosterone and angiotensin II are the two effector compounds in this system that act directly on tissues. Potassium and adrenocorticotropic hormone (ACTH) stimulate aldosterone secretion, as does angiotensin II, while large increases in plasma sodium concentration inhibit aldosterone release.

The main clinical use for measurement of components of the renin-angiotensin system is for the diagnosis of secondary hypertension. Patients with primary aldosteronism have suppressed plasma renin activity, and measurement of differential renal vein renin activity in patients with renovascular lesions helps to predict the outcome of surgery, although not with complete accuracy.[146]

If plasma renin activity is measured in a group of normal subjects of comparable age, under standard conditions of posture, activity, diet, and time of day, values will be found to fall within a relatively narrow range, especially if the measurements are made in the controlled environment of a metabolic study ward. Outpatient studies offer less precision because it is difficult for an outpatient to adhere to a constant metabolic diet. An attempt has been made to solve this difficulty by taking advantage of the fact that plasma renin activity reflects recent sodium intake. Thus, Brunner and his co-workers collected a 24-hour urine sample for measurement of sodium excretion on the day that blood was drawn for measurement of plasma renin activity, after their subjects had been up and about for the morning[147] (see Fig 5–8). Other investigators have subdivided patients on the basis of plasma renin activity after administration of a diuretic.[148] Drayer has found that plasma renin activity after 5 days of chlorthalidone therapy provides an accurate and inexpensive way to characterize patients.[149]

When one measures renin activity in patients with essential hypertension, the values spread over a much wider range than are seen in normal subjects. Roughly 30% of the patients will have renin activity lower than normal, and around 10%–15% will have activity higher than normal. Thus, patients with essential hypertension can be subdivided on the basis of high, normal, or low plasma renin activity. After several years of intensive research, the cause of low-renin hypertension is not clear.[150] The physiology of renin release suggests that patients with low-renin hypertension might be relatively volume overloaded, as are patients with primary aldosteronism; while those with high renin activity might be volume depleted and relatively vasoconstricted because of high circulating angiotensin II levels, as is found in patients with malignant or renovascular hypertension. Thus, concepts of "volume-dependent" or low-renin hypertension, and "vasoconstrictor-dependent" or high-renin hypertension, have evolved.[151] As shown in Table 5–1, most types of hypertension can be classified in this manner.

TABLE 5–1.—ANGIOTENSIN II GENERATION IN HYPERTENSIVE
VASCULAR DISEASE*

LOW PLASMA RENIN ACTIVITY	NORMAL PLASMA RENIN ACTIVITY	HIGH PLASMA RENIN ACTIVITY

A. Aldosteronism
  1. Primary
  2. Pseudoprimary
  3. Tertiary?
  4. Glucocorticoid suppressible
B. Mineralocorticoidism
  1. 11-β hydroxylase deficiency
  2. 17-α hydroxylase deficiency
  3. Adrenal carcinoma
  4. Ectopic ACTH-secreting tumors
  5. Excess 18-OH DOC?
C. Not clearly demonstrable
  1. Low-renin essential hypertension
  2. Parenchymal renal disease†
  3. Liddle's syndrome
  4. Gordon's hyperkalemic patient
  5. Iatrogenic: mineralocorticoid or licorice ingestion
	A. Normal aldosterone secretion
	  1. Normal-renin essential hypertension
	  2. Unilateral renal disease†
	  3. Bilateral renal vascular or parenchymal disease†
	  4. Cushing's syndrome
	  5. Coarctation of the aorta
	  6. Pheochromocytoma
		A. Secondary aldosteronism
		  1. Malignant or severe hypertension
		  2. Unilateral renal disease with severe hypertension
		  3. Bilateral renal vascular or parenchymal disease†
		  4. High renin essential hypertension
		  5. Renin-secreting kidney tumors
		  6. Iatrogenic: oral contraceptive use
		B. Without secondary aldosteronism
		  1. Potassium depleted patients with above disorders

*From Laragh, J.H., et al.: Renin, angiotensin and aldosterone systems in pathogenesis and management of hypertensive vascular disease. *Am. J. Med.* 52:633, 1972. Used by permission.
†Note that patients with parenchymal or renal vascular (unilateral or bilateral) disease may exhibit low, normal, or high circulating plasma renin activity.

The effect of various antihypertensive agents have been studied in low-renin hypertension to test the hypothesis that blood pressure elevation in such patients is volume-dependent. Most workers now agree that these patients respond well to aminoglutethimide, which blocks the synthesis of mineralocorticoids[152] to thiazide diuretics[151] or to spironolactone, an aldosterone antagonist.[153]

Patients with high-renin hypertension have been treated with propranolol, a β-adrenergic blocking agent that blocks the release of renin. It has been reported that patients with high-renin hypertension respond unusually well to this form of therapy but the observation remains controversial.[141] Woods and his co-workers have examined this problem with a prospective, double-blind crossover study of 54 patients with low- and normal-renin essential hypertension.[154] The patients were classified by three methods: upright plasma renin activity versus 24-hour urinary sodium excretion on an ad lib. diet; plasma renin activity after furosemide diuresis and upright posture; and plasma renin activity after 7 days on a 65-mEq sodium diet versus 24-hour sodium excretion. Although a good correlation was found among the methods, the three did not exactly identify the same patients with low renin activity. All patients then received chlorthalidone for 18 weeks, then propranolol for 18 weeks, or vice versa. Chlorthalidone was found to lower blood pressure more effectively than propranolol in a daily dose of 3.5 mg/kg/day. As a group, low-renin patients had no greater reduction of pressure after receiving chlorthalidone than did normal-renin patients. Also, patients with normal-renin hypertension did not have a greater reduction in blood pressure in response to propranolol than did patients with low-renin hypertension. However, when the distribution of blood pressure responses within the groups was analyzed, it was found that chlorthalidone reduced blood pressure to normal in a larger percentage of patients with either low or normal plasma renin activity than did propranolol and that chlorthalidone was particularly effective in the low-renin group. The authors concluded that renin measurements were of limited benefit in selecting antihypertension therapy and recommended initiating therapy with diuretics in the usual patient.

Roughly one third of patients with essential hypertension have low-renin, or volume-dependent hypertension, and another 60% have normal renin activity, which suggests that they, too, have a volume component to their blood pressure problem. Thus, 80%–90% of patients with hypertension might be expected to respond to diuretic therapy. Those patients who fail to respond to diuretics are ordinarily placed on sympatholytic drugs, which tend to decrease renin release.[155] Thus, a conventional therapeutic approach will eventually cover the spectrum of high- to low-renin hypertension.

Compounds have been developed which either block converting enzyme activity, thus preventing the formation of angiotensin II (teprotide, a nonapeptide),[156] captopril,[157] enalapril,[158] and lisinopril,[159] or which block angiotensin II receptors (saralasin, a synthetic octapeptide).[160] These agents, used sequentially with diuretics, allow more precise estimation of the relative contribution of the renal pressor system and that of effective blood volume to the production of hypertension in a given patient. For example, intravenous infusion of saralasin or a converting enzyme inhibitor will be followed by a drop in blood pressure if the patient has a renin-dependent form of hypertension. The administration of a diuretic then reveals the contribution of the volume component in part, but this contribution is masked by reactive hyperreninemia caused by the administration of the diuretic. If the blocking compound is then given a second time, the contribution of effective blood volume can then be assessed.[161] These agents have been found to be useful in identifying patients with renovascular hypertension.[162] Plasma renin activity has also been found to play a role in the antihypertensive effect of calcium channel blockers; patients with low renin activity show a more pronounced reduction in blood pressure than patients whose renin activity is relatively high.[161]

PROSTAGLANDINS AND THE KALLIKREIN-KININ SYSTEM

Contained within the cardiovascular system are several control points at which disorders of prostaglandin metabolism might contribute to alterations in blood pressure. In addition, the prostaglandins play an important role in the regulation of uterine blood flow during pregnancy and may be involved in the etiology of preeclampsia-eclampsia. As mentioned earlier, elevated blood pressure reflects a disturbed relationship between cardiac output and peripheral vascular resistance, and patients with uncomplicated essential hypertension usually have a normal cardiac output and an elevated vascular resistance. The interplay of intrinsic and extrinsic factors in the control of resistance offers multiple sites for interactions with prostaglandins that might disturb blood pressure regulation either by an excess of prohypertensive factors or by inadequate antihypertensive influences.

Total peripheral resistance is influenced by several blood-borne substances; e.g., vasoconstriction can be amplified by circulating angiotensin II or catecholamines. As prostaglandins function primarily as local hormones, they oppose the actions of circulating hormones by virtue of their synthesis at the site of action of the circulating hormone in vascular smooth muscle.

An alternative mechanism which affects vascular resistance is local release of norepinephrine from nerve endings, which results in vasoconstriction. Local release of norepinephrine is an important component of the overall integrated function of the central nervous system in circulatory control. Local production of prostaglandin E_2 (PGE$_2$) influences vascular tone by interfering with release of norepinephrine from nerve endings.[163] Genetic or environmental influences which could impair local PGE$_2$ or prostaglandin I_2 (PGI$_2$) production, or accelerated destruction of these compounds, might account for the enhanced vascular reactivity known to occur in the earliest phases of essential hypertension.

There are three intrinsic mechanisms important in the regulation of vascular resistance:[12] basal vascular tone, the Bayliss effect,[13] and, perhaps most important relative to the production of prostaglandins, the influence of local tissue metabolites on vascular resistance. As tissue perfusion falls, oxygen delivery becomes inadequate, local adenosine triphosphate (ATP) breakdown exceeds synthesis, and a number of vasodilator substances accumulate. Which compound, if any, bears the greatest influence on local autoregulation has not been established. It is at this point that prostaglandins undoubtedly exert an important effect on overall circulatory regulation. Local production of PGI$_2$ and of PGE$_2$ would result in vasodilatation, while production of thromboxane A_2 and prostaglandin F_2 (PGF$_2$) would contribute to vasoconstriction.

The other major component in the regulation of blood pressure is cardiac output. Young patients with labile hypertension often have a hyperkinetic circulation characterized by a high cardiac output.[48] Although this finding has been attributed to overactivity of the sympathetic nervous system, it is conceivable that deficient prostaglandin synthesis, or increased destruction, would remove their modulating effect on norepinephrine release, thus resulting in a higher heart rate, which could contribute to an increased cardiac output as well as an inadequate fall in vascular resistance.

The prostaglandins are potentially important in regulating both myocardial preload and afterload. Increased production of prostaglandin $F_{2\alpha}$ ($PGF_{2\alpha}$), a venoconstrictor,[164] would result in increased venous return and a subsequent increase in cardiac output. The vasodilator effects of PGI_2 and PGE_2 would decrease afterload and might contribute to decreased preload by dilating veins. On the other hand, the vasoconstrictor effect of $PGF_{2\alpha}$ and of thromboxane A_2 may increase both preload and afterload.

In experimental animals, prostaglandins have variable effects on myocardial contractility, depending upon experimental conditions and species. Most studies have shown that prostaglandins of the E and A series increase cardiac output and have a positive inotropic effect.[165] In man, infusions of PGE_1 increase stroke volume and heart rate, thus increasing cardiac output; this gives rise to the hypothesis that excess synthesis of prostaglandins of the E series contributes to a hyperkinetic circulatory state, which in turn may initiate a chain of events leading to hypertension.[166] Blood pressure also depends upon the volume of blood contained within the vascular tree. A large body of evidence now links renal prostaglandin metabolism to the regulation and distribution of renal bood flow.

Siren[167] studied the central actions of arachidonic acid and $PGF_{2\alpha}$ in the spontaneously hypertensive rat and found that intraventricular administration of either compound resulted in an increase in blood pressure, heart rate, and temperature in both normal and hypertensive animals. However, the magnitude of the blood pressure response was greater in the spontaneously hypertensive rat.

Prostaglandins and Blood Vessels

The mechanisms by which prostaglandins influence peripheral vascular resistance fall into three general categories. First, peripheral vascular resistance is influenced by the vasodilating or vasoconstricting effects of locally synthesized prostaglandins,[168] e.g., PGE_2, PGI_2, and $PGF_{2\alpha}$. The second mechanism is modulation, by locally synthesized vasoactive compounds, of the actions of other substances. For example, locally synthesized PGE_2 impairs release of norepinephrine from nerve terminals.[163] Third, peripheral vascular resistance is indirectly affected by prostaglandins synthesized elsewhere; e.g., synthesis of PGE_2 is important in maintaining renal blood flow, particularly to the inner cortex and medulla.[169] Prostaglandins also play a role in salt and water excretion; the latter is accomplished in part by interfering with the action of ADH on the collecting tubules.[170] Prostaglandins synthesized in the kidney, therefore, can influence total body sodium and water, thus influencing plasma and intracellular fluid volume and sodium balance and, thereby, the reactivity of vascular smooth muscle to pressor agents.

Recent studies suggest that PGI_2 is released into the circulation from the pulmonary vascular bed.[171, 172] Unlike other prostaglandins, PGI_2 is not destroyed during passage through the lungs[173, 174] and could influence peripheral arteriolar tone. Prostaglandin A_2 (PGA_2), when infused intravenously, is not destroyed during passage through the pulmonary circulation,[175] causes vasodilatation, natriuresis, and diuresis, and has an antihypertensive effect.[176] Early studies suggested that PGA_2 was released from the kidney in response to sodium deprivation, thus functioning as a systemic hormone.[177] More recent studies, which were based on highly sensitive and specific mass spectrometric methods for the measurement of PGA_2 failed to confirm its presence in circulating blood.[178, 179]

Piper and Vane[180] reported that one or more substances that were released from guinea pig lung during anaphylaxis contracted the rabbit aorta. Later, it was found that indomethacin blocked the formation of "rabbit aorta contracting material" (RCS), suggesting that RCS might be related to a precursor of prostaglandins. The eventual discovery of the endoperoxides, and their isolation in pure form, enabled them to be distinguished from RCS by their longer half-life in aqueous solution. In a series of experiments involving the synthesis of prostaglandins in blood platelets, Hamberg and Samuelsson[181] found that endoperoxides within platelets are converted into a hemiacetal derivative with an oxane structure, plus malondialdehyde and a C17-hydroxy acid (Fig 5–9). The first compound, now designated thromboxane B_2, is the breakdown product of A_2, an unstable intermediate. Formed in platelets and in other tissues subjected to injury, thromboxane A_2 contributes to platelet aggregation and produces vasoconstriction[182] and may be involved in the genesis of disseminated intravascular coagulation and of vasospasm which characterize preeclampsia-eclampsia.

Bunting et al.[183] have demonstrated another unstable product of the transformation of the endoperoxides. The structure of this substance has been elucidated, and the compound has been designated PGI_2, or prostacyclin. This compound, which is produced by blood vessels, has two important biologic effects, vasodilatation and inhibition of platelet

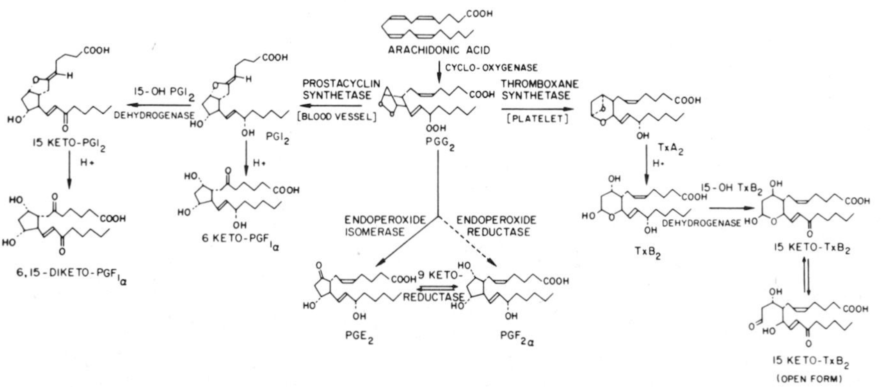

Fig 5–9.—Metabolism of arachidonic acid by the prostaglandin synthetase complex. A major product of vascular tissues is prostacyclin *(PGI$_2$)* and a major product of blood platelets is thromboxane A$_2$ *(TxA$_2$)*. (From Sullivan J.M., McGiff J.C.: Kallikrein-kinin and prostaglandin systems in hypertension, in Rosenthal J. (ed.): *Arterial Hypertension, Pathogenesis, Diagnosis and Therapy.* New York, Springer-Verlag, New York, 1982. Used by permission.)

aggregation. Moncada et al.[184] have demonstrated that vascular rings from human colic or gastric blood vessels will synthesize PGI$_2$, and the veins will produce more PGI$_2$ than the arteries do. The effect occurs spontaneously but disappears with time or with washing of the specimens. Incubation of washed vascular tissue with arachidonate then restores production of prostacyclin. This production can be blocked in two ways: first, by the addition of indomethacin, which, by inhibiting cyclooxygenase, prevents the conversion of arachidonic acid into endoperoxides; and the second, by the addition of 15-hydroxy-peroxyarachidonic acid, which blocks the conversion of endoperoxides to prostacyclin by inhibiting the prostacyclin synthetase step.

The addition of prostacyclin-synthesizing vascular rings to platelet-rich plasma inhibits platelet aggregation. It is possible that endothelial production of prostacyclin is the mechanism by which the body prevents thrombus formation throughout the healthy vascular tree. Vascular tissue that is injured either by trauma, such as abrupt elevation of blood pressure during pregnancy, or by atherosclerosis might not be able to synthesize prostacyclin adequately, thus allowing the deposition of platelets, formation of thrombi, and perhaps initiation or acceleration of atherosclerosis. It can also be postulated that failure to synthesize might result in elevated vascular resistance.

As noted previously, local synthesis of PGE$_2$ in the vessel wall can interfere with adrenergic transmission, primarily by inhibiting the release of norepinephrine from nerve terminals.[163] This would result in vasodilatation, or at least diminished vasoconstriction, thus playing a potentially important role in local or systemic regulation of blood flow and pressure. In addition, local synthesis of PGE_2 and PGI_2 in vascular walls antagonizes the effect of both norepinephrine and angiotensin II and may play a role in angiotensin tachyphylaxis. Aiken[185] used femoral and celiac arterial strips to study the effects of angiotensin II. Doses repeated every 30 minutes continued to contract the femoral strips but had progressively less effect on the celiac artery strips. When inhibitors of cyclooxygenase were given, tachyphylaxis did not develop in the celiac strips. The addition of PGE_2 had no effect on the contraction of femoral arterial strips evoked by angiotensin II but reduced the effect of angiotensin II on the celiac arterial strips. The experiments of Aiken[185] suggested that angiotensin II can stimulate and release prostaglandins in the vascular wall, thus blunting its own vasoconstrictor effect, at least in the mesenteric vascular bed. Angiotensin II has been reported to stimulate the release of PGI_2 from the kidney,[186] the lung, blood vessels,[187] and the heart.[188] These observations may explain the loss of sensitivity to angiotensin II that takes place in normal pregnancy. Both PGE_2 and PGI_2 have been shown to attenuate the pressor responses to norepinephrine[189] and to angiotensin II.[190] Thus, failure of an organ to synthesize adequate amounts of PGE_2 or PGI_2 in response to a pressor stimulus is a potential mechanism for the development of elevated vascular resistance and hypertension.[190]

A number of attempts have been made to produce hypertension by treating experimental animals with inhibitors of cyclooxygenase. These experiments have yielded conflicting results. Beilin and Bhattacharya[191] and Colina-Chourio et al.[192] observed an elevation of blood pressure in rabbits treated with indomethacin, while Muirhead et al.[193] did not. Romero and Strong[194] administered indomethacin to rabbits with one-clip, two-kidney renovascular hypertension and found no effect on blood pressure in rabbits with normal renal blood flow and normal plasma renin activity, whereas hypertension was aggravated in animals with low renal blood flow and elevated plasma renin activity. Although plasma renin activity initially fell in both groups, it did not stay suppressed in those animals whose blood pressure increased. Thus, in the rabbit, indomethacin appears to exert at least a dual effect on blood pressure, one through suppression of renin release and the other through an effect on resistance vessels. In the rat[195, 196, 197] and in the dog,[198] similarly conflicting results have been obtained.

The systemic hemodynamic effects of inhibited prostaglandin synthesis were studied in man by Wennmalm.[199] Six normal subjects underwent arterial cannulation and right heart catheterization. Blood pressure and cardiac output were measured before and after intravenous administration of 25 mg of indomethacin. Diastolic blood pressure rose by 16% and systemic vascular resistance rose by 49%. Nowak and Wennmalm[200] have found that the chronic administration of indomethacin to normal subjects results in a modest elevation of blood pressure, while others have failed to produce such an elevation.[201] Patak et al.[202] have reported that indomethacin aggravated hypertension in man and antagonized the effects of furosemide. Durao et al.[203] have observed that indomethacin counteracted the antihypertensive effects of both pindolol and propranolol in 7 hypertensive patients who had previously been controlled by β-blockade. In view of current knowledge, several explanations are possible. Intravenously administered indomethacin might have prevented the formation of vascular PGE_2 or PGI_2 thereby allowing vasoconstriction to take place unimpeded by the modulating influence of the prostaglandins, or the inhibiting effects of PGE_2 on norepinephrine release might have been removed, allowing adrenergically induced vasoconstriction to take place. Another mechanism is suggested by the observations of De Jong et al.,[204] who noted that indomethacin actually lowered blood pressure in two siblings with renin-dependent hypertension, while also lowering plasma renin activity and plasma aldosterone concentration. These studies point to an important role for the prostaglandin system in the regulation of blood pressure in man. However, the conflicting reports indicate that the matter requires additional investigation.

With the information that blood vessels have the capacity to synthesize two compounds with potentially important antihypertensive effects, it is a logical step to apply the model of an enzyme deficiency disease and propose that hypertension might follow inadequate synthesis of either PGI_2 or PGE_2. However, when this hypothesis has been examined in spontaneously hypertensive animals, or animals that are made hypertensive by renal artery constriction or the administration of deoxycorticosterone acetate (DOCA) and salt, the opposite has been found to be the case, i.e., while blood pressure was elevated, increased prostaglandin synthesis has been found.

Rioux et al.[205] have studied the release of prostaglandin-like material from the aortas of normal rats, spontaneously hypertensive rats (SHR), and rats in whom hypertension had been induced, either by renal artery constriction or by administration of DOCA and salt. Increased release of prostaglandins was observed in all three forms of hypertension. Furthermore, prostaglandin release returned to normal levels when hypertension was reversed in the rats whose hypertension had been induced. Similarly, Limas and Limas[206] have observed increased levels of prostaglandin synthetase activity in the microsomal fraction of the renal medulla of SHRs. More recently, Pace-Asciak et al.[207] found that aortic rings and homogenates from SHRs had an increased ability to convert arachidonic acid to PGI_2 suggesting impaired synthesis of a vasodilating compound.

Pipili and Poyser[208] found that the output of PGI_2 from the mesenteric arterial bed of the hypertensive rats was higher than that of normotensive animals. Sympathetic nerve stimulation increased PGI_2 release from the mesenteric bed of the normotensive rat but not from the hypertensive rat.

Data are emerging that indicate that local production of prostaglandins, mainly PGI_2, plays an important role in the regulation of local vascular resistance. Several studies have shown that blockade of prostaglandin synthesis in the kidney results in a reduction in the concentration of prostaglandin-like material in renal venous blood and a fall in total renal blood flow.[209, 210, 211] Studies of the effect of blockade of prostaglandin synthesis on blood flow in extremities have yielded conflicting results. Aiken and Vane[210] found no significant increase in hindlimb vascular resistance in the dog hindlimb after treatment with indomethacin. However, Lonigro et al.[211] and Beaty and Donald[212] have found that treatment with indomethacin or meclofenamate was followed by an increase in resting vascular resistance in the dog hindlimb. Beaty and Donald[212] further noted that the blockade of prostaglandin synthesis had no effect on blood flow in the exercising hindlimb, but it did have an effect on reactive hyperemia, which progressively diminished the longer the vascular occlusion was maintained. This suggests that the local accumulation of metabolites during exercise, or in tissues distal to a vascular occlusion, was capable of overriding the relative vasoconstriction that occurred when prostaglandin synthesis was blocked.

Ishii et al.[213] have studied plasma levels of 6-keto-prostaglandin $F_{1\alpha}$ (6-keto-$PGF_{1\alpha}$) in normal subjects and in patients with essential hypertension and have compared the effect of intravenous infusions of norepinephrine on hemodynamics and 6-keto-$PGF_{1\alpha}$ levels. They found reduced levels of 6-keto-$PGF_{1\alpha}$ in the plasma of essential hypertensive patients. In response to norepinephrine, the normal subjects increased both cardiac index and total peripheral resistance, while in the patients with essential hypertension only cardiac output increased. Norepinephrine infusion resulted in an increase in plasma levels of 6-keto-$PGF_{1\alpha}$ that was greater in normal subjects than in the patients with hypertension. Ishii and his co-workers concluded that prostaglandin metabolism was altered in patients with essential hypertension.

Chaignon et al.[214] have studied the effect of intravenous infusions of prostaglandin I_2 in patients with severe hypertension. Treatment with PGI_2 decreased mean blood pressure from 154 to 120 mm Hg and decreased total peripheral resistance by 45%. Concomitantly, cardiac index rose 40%. Plasma norepinephrine and plasma renin activity also increased during PGI_2 infusions. Measurements of blood volumes during PGI_2 infusions revealed a central translocation of blood. Thus, PGI_2 is an effective vasodilator that lowers blood pressure, but the antihypertensive effect is blunted by the increase in cardiac output.

Lima and Turner[215] have studied the effect of prostacyclin on lymphocyte adenosine 3′:5′-cyclic phosphate (cyclic-AMP) production before and after β-blockade with propranolol. They found that prior treatment with a β-blocking agent significantly increased the amount of prostacyclin-induced cyclic-AMP production and suggested that prostaglandin causes vasodilatation of vascular beds during β-adrenergic blockade, thus contributing to the antihypertensive effect.

The Blood Platelets and Prostaglandins

As knowledge of the pathways of prostaglandin metabolism has evolved, it has become apparent that compounds having different ac-

Fig 5–10.—Cross section of the vascular wall showing possible interactions of prostaglandins and vasoactive hormones. Magnification of the vascular wall, interfaced with blood and a circulating platelet, is shown at the lower portion of the figure. At the endothelial surface and the subendothelial zone of vascular tissues, the major product of arachidonic acid *(AA)* metabolism arising from tissue stores of phospholipids *(PL)* is prostacyclin *(PGI₂)*. A major product of arachidonic acid metabolism within the aggregating platelet is thromboxane A₂ *(TxA₂)*. Formation of thromboxane A₂ within the vasculature may occur only under pathologic conditions. Angiotensin and bradykinin, which activate acylhydrolases within the vascular wall, promote prostaglandin synthesis. In addition to PGI₂, *PGE₂* is a major product of arachidonic acid metabolism in the vascular wall. Its main function may be to modulate release of the adrenergic neurotransmitter, norepinephrine *(NE)*. Further, PGE₂ may be converted to *PGF₂ₐ* on activation of the enzyme PGE-9-ketoreductase by either angiotensin or bradykinin.

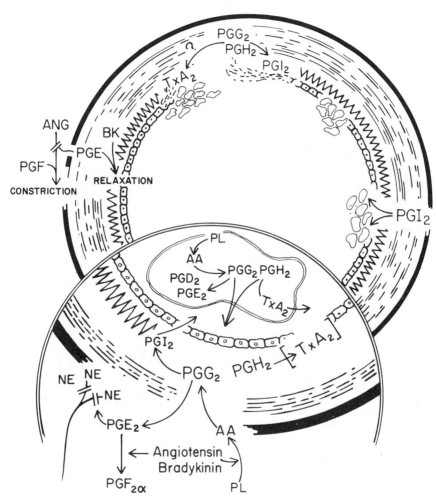

Outside the area of magnification, additional interactions of prostaglandins are shown. On the right, the formation of PGI_2 repels aggregating platelets. At the top, the failure of formation of PGI_2 in an area of damaged endothelium results in platelet aggregation which may be related to the evolution of atherosclerosis. Upon injury of vascular tissues, formation of PGI_2 may be comprised, and thromboxane A_2 formation, both by platelets and vascular tissue, may predominate *(top)*. On the left, possible interactions of angiotensin *(ANG)* and bradykinin *(BK)* with prostaglandins are indicated: PGE_2 may contribute to the vasodilator effects of bradykinin *(relaxation)*. In contrast, PGE_2 usually antagonizes the vasoconstrictor effect of angiotensin, whereas $PGF_{2\alpha}$ may facilitate this action of angiotensin. (From Sullivan J.M., McGiff J.C.: Kallikrein-kinin and prostaglandin systems in hypertension, in Rosenthal J. (ed.): *Arterial Hypertension, Pathogenesis, Diagnosis and Therapy.* New York, Springer-Verlag, New York, 1982.)

tions are synthesized from the same precursors in blood vessels and in blood platelets; and these products of the endoperoxides, thromboxane A_2 of platelets, and prostacyclin of vascular tissues, play counterbalancing roles (Fig 5–10). In the blood vessel wall, conversion of the cyclic endoperoxides into prostacyclin results in the formation of a product that prevents platelet aggregation and promotes vasodilatation.[184] On the other hand, in the aggregating platelet the endoperoxides prostaglandin G_2 (PGG_2) and prostaglandin H_2 (PGH_2) are converted largely to thromboxane A_2, a potent vasoconstrictor whose formation is associated with platelet aggregation. This compound, thromboxane A_2, has a half life in aqueous solution of only 30 seconds and is a vasoconstrictor.[182]

Both aspirin and indomethacin inhibit cyclooxygenase activity, thus preventing the conversion of arachidonic acid to endoperoxides, and thereby their breakdown products, thromboxane A_2, PGI_2, and PGE_2. A clinical observation has confirmed the importance of this pathway and has provided the first definite evidence for a biologic role of the prostaglandins. Malmsten et al.[216] have reported a patient with a bleeding disorder due to congenital deficiency of platelet cyclooxygenase. The platelets from this subject contained normal stores of adenosine diphosphate but showed impaired aggregation in response to collagen, epinephrine, or arachidonic acid; yet, the platelets aggregated in response to PGG_2. Studies with radiolabeled arachidonic acid proved that the patient's platelets failed to form endoperoxides.

Despite thromboxane A_2's potency as a vasoconstrictor, there is no evidence to date that this compound is present in circulating plasma or that enhanced release of thromboxane contributes to elevated vascular resistance in any experimental model. There is evidence that PGI_2 is released into the circulation after synthesis in the vasculature of the lung. Gryglewski et al.[171] and Moncada et al.[172] have shown that arterial blood contains an unstable disaggregating substance that enhances the effect of exogenous PGI_2 and is present in greater amounts in arterial than in venous blood. While this substance may serve to reduce platelet aggregation during turbulent flow in a high pressure system, impaired release might also be associated with increased vascular resistance. This area remains speculative, however, since vascular tissues have been reported to contain sufficient prostaglandin dehydrogenase activity to inactivate PGI_2 within the vessel wall.[217]

Whether or not PGI_2 functions as a circulating hormone remains a matter for additional investigation. Several observations support the conclusion that PGI_2 is released from the pulmonary endothelium into the pulmonary capillary circulation. Hensby et al.[218] have demonstrated higher concentrations of 6-oxo-prostaglandin $F_{1\alpha}$, a breakdown product of PGI_2, in the left ventricle than in the pulmonary arteries of 5 human subjects. Recent evidence supports the concept that a breakdown product of PGI_2 might mediate some of PGI_2's properties. Szczeklik et al.[219] demonstrated that both blood pressure and platelet response to ADP were suppressed for one hour after inhalation of PGI_2, far exceeding the known half-life of PGI_2 in blood, which is 2 to 3 minutes. Gimeno et al.[220] and Hoult et al.[221] have presented evidence that PGI_2 is transferred by plasma or blood platelets into a product with bioactivity similar to 6-keto-PGE_1. Wong et al.[222] have recovered 9-hydroxy prostaglandin dehydrogenase (9-OH PGDH) from the cytoplasm of human platelets that metabolized the methyl ester of PGI_2 to (22-3H)-6-keto-PGE_1 methyl ester. Intact platelets effected the same conversion, demonstrating that the PGI_2 has access to the cytosolic enzyme. Since 6-keto-PGF_1 is stable and has platelet inhibiting properties, it is possible that this compound accounts for the reduced platelet aggregation found in arterial blood.

Prostaglandins and the Kidney

There are a number of ways the kidney participates in the regulation of blood pressure. Malfunction of one or both might lead to elevated blood pressure. First, the kidney plays a pivotal role in the regulation of extracellular fluid volume. In addition to excretion of fluid, the kidney is also involved in the regulation of electrolyte balance. Retention of sodium leads to enhanced vascular responsiveness to pressor stimuli.[223] Potassium depletion results in impaired dilatation, which in turn might lead to hypertension.[224] The kidney releases pressor substances that affect vascular resistance. Angiotensin I may function as a vasoconstricting agent within the kidney;[225] it is converted to the pressor angiotensin II primarily during passage across the lungs.[226] The kidney also produces antihypertensive substances, such as vasodepressor neutral lipids[227] and prostaglandins.[228]

As prostaglandins are involved in the regulation of renal function, evidence linking prostaglandin synthesis and degradation to hypertension has been sought. However, the evidence derived from experiments using surgically or pharmacologically induced hypertension in animals has questionable relevance to human hypertension, and studies of spontaneously hypertensive rats have yielded conflicting results. For example, Dunn[229] and Limas and Limas[206] have found increased prostaglandin synthetase activity in the renal medullae of spontaneously hypertensive rats, while Pace-Asciak[230] and Limas and Limas[206] have found decreased 15-prostaglandin dehydrogenase activity, which degrades prostaglandins, in the renal cortex of SHRs, and Stygles et al.[231] found no change in renal PGE_2 production in the renomedullary tissues of SHRs, even after the development of hypertension. Ahnfelt-Rønne and Arrigoni-Martelli[232] have found evidence of increased $PGF_{2\alpha}$ synthesis in the renal papillae of Wistar-Kyoto-Okamoto rats, while Armstrong et al.[233] have not found this to be the case in New Zealand SHRs. In studies of human subjects with essential hypertension, Tan et al.[234] found evidence of impaired renal production of prostaglandin E_2, which, through reduction of renal blood flow and retention of sodium and water, could result in elevated blood pressure.

Prostaglandins play a role in the regulation of renal blood flow, particularly when renal function is challenged.[169, 235] McGiff et al.[236] showed that antidiuresis and renal vasoconstriction evoked by angiotensin II were diminished due to intrarenal release of PGE_2, the principal product of prostaglandin synthesis in the kidney that can attenuate the action of antidiuretic hormone.[170] Later, Aiken and Vane[210] showed that indomethacin administration resulted in enhanced vasoconstrictor effects of angiotensin II in the kidney.

Inhibition of prostaglandin cyclooxygenase results in reduction of all products formed downstream from this step (see Fig 5–9). Not only is production of the vasodilator and natriuretic agent, PGE_2, diminished, but also that of the vasoconstrictor, $PGF_{2\alpha}$. Synthesis of PGI_2 and thromboxane A_2 is also inhibited.[183] Experiments using either indomethacin, meclofenamate, aspirin, ibuprofen, or other nonsteroidal anti-inflammatory agents result in diminished production of all the products of arachidonic acid metabolism, which have markedly different physiologic effects. Therefore, the effects of cyclooxygenase inhibitors on the renal circulation vary widely with experimental conditions. Terragno et al.[169] have shown that indomethacin does not affect renal blood flow in either the anesthetized or conscious dog. However, when the anesthetized dog is acutely stressed by laparotomy, a large increase in renal prostaglandin release occurs. Under these conditions, administration of indomethacin greatly increases renal vascular resistance and renal venous prostaglandin levels fall to those observed in the conscious dog. Any stress will increase prostaglandin release several-fold. This increase is associated with maintenance of renal blood flow at normal levels. When indomethacin is administered under these conditions, a precipitous decrease in renal blood flow results.

A prostaglandin-dependent mechanism is involved not only in the regulation of renal blood flow during stress but also in the intrarenal distribution of blood flow. In studies using the isolated dog kidney, Itskovitz et al.[237] found that blood levels of PGE_2 correlated with increased fractional blood flow to the inner cortex, while indomethacin caused a disproportionate reduction of blood flow to the inner cortex, which resulted in a redistribution of renal blood flow. A possible clinical correlation of these findings is the nephropathy of analgesic abuse. This condition has been suggested to be due to medullary ischemia secondary to reduced synthesis of one or more vasodilator prostaglandins. However, the capacity to synthesize prostaglandins is shared by a number of structures in all zones of the kidney. Larsson and Anggard[238] have demonstrated synthesis of prostaglandins in the renal cortex. Cyclooxygenase is known to be present in three different tissues in the kidney. The interstitial cells of the renal medulla have the ability to synthesize prostaglandins,[227] as do the vascular structures of the kidney,[239] and the cells lining the distal nephron and collecting ducts.[240] The latter location accords with the known interrelationships between prostaglandins and ADH. Antidiuretic hormone causes a greater concentration of urinary solute if given after treatment with indomethacin.[241] Thus a prostaglandin of the E series blunts the effects of ADH[170] and favors the excretion of free water.[241]

Tobian et al.[242] have reported reduced levels of PGE_2 in the renal papillae of Dahl salt-sensitive rats and further noted that salt loading resulted in a lesser increase in PGE_2 than was observed in Dahl salt-resistant rats. By feeding Dahl S rats a diet high in linoleic acid, a precursor of arachidonic acid, Tobian and his co-workers[242] were able to restore renal PGE_2 levels to normal and to prevent the sodium-related increase in blood pressure.

Interrelationship of Prostaglandins and the Renin-Angiotensin System

The prostaglandin and the renin-angiotensin-aldosterone systems have complex interrelationships. Infusion of angiotensin II results in release of renal prostaglandins.[236] Arachidonic acid, the precursor of renal prostaglandins, enhances renin release.[131] Indomethacin decreases plasma renin activity and prevents the effects of arachidonic acid. Indomethacin also prevents prostaglandin release in response to angiotensin. Thus, a prostaglandin mechanism appears to participate in the regulation of renin release, while generation of angiotensin following release of renin can in turn stimulate prostaglandin synthesis. Frölich et al.[243] have studied prostaglandin mechanisms in the regulation of plasma renin activity in man. They found that indomethacin administration is followed by diminished plasma renin activity, plasma aldosterone concentration, and urinary sodium and prostaglandin excretion in both normal and hypertensive subjects. As angiotensin infusion continues to stimulate aldosterone secretion after the administration of indomethacin, the effect of the indomethacin on aldosterone secretion is due presumably to diminished generation of angiotensin. They have also noted that indomethacin prevents the immediate increase in plasma renin activity that ordinarily follows administration of furosemide. Indomethacin has two effects that might explain these observations. First, it interferes with the synthesis of prostaglandins. Secondly, indomethacin causes sodium and fluid retention. Thus, the relative contribution of inhibition of prostaglandin synthesis and of sodium retention to the fall in plasma renin activity that ordinarily follows indomethacin administration is not clear.

Weber et al.[244] have demonstrated that PGE_2, the principal product of renal prostaglandin synthesis, did not directly affect renin release from renal slices. However, a metabolic intermediate in the production of PGE_2, the endoperoxide PGG_2, was shown to increase renin release. These data suggest that inhibition of PGE_2 synthesis does not affect renin release directly; rather, the suppression of prostaglandin endoperoxide synthesis, or one of its breakdown products, may be the determining factor. Whorton et al.[245] have demonstrated the release of renin from rabbit renal cortical slices incubated with PGI_2. A linear response was observed over 30 minutes of incubation, which suggested that a breakdown product of PGI_2 might be involved, in view of the short half-life of PGI_2, in aqueous solution. However, the hydrolysis product of PGI_2, 6-keto-$PGF_{1\alpha}$, was not active. Hoult and Moore[246] have subsequently found 9-hydroxyprostaglandin dehydrogenase (9-OH PGDH) activity in the kidney, the product of which, 6-keto-PGE_1, is stable and has been demonstrated to be a potent stimulator of renin release by Spokas et al.[247] Jackson et al.[248] have examined renin secretion rates after infusion of either PGI_2 or 6-keto-PGE_2 into the renal artery of the dog and found 6-keto-PGE$_1$ to be five times more potent than PGI$_2$.

The relationship between prostaglandin synthesis and plasma renin activity has important implications in the treatment of patients with Bartter's syndrome.[249] Although this syndrome is not associated with hypertension, it is a clinical example of an association between a disorder of vascular reactivity and prostaglandin metabolism. Bartter's syndrome is characterized by renal juxtaglomerular hyperplasia, elevation of plasma renin activity, plasma angiotensin II concentration and aldosterone secretory rate, hypokalemic alkalosis, normal blood pressure, and resistance to the pressor effects of angiotensin II and norepinephrine. These features resemble a normal pregnancy and may point to an explanation of the mechanisms of hemodynamic adaptation to normal pregnancy. The renal tubular reabsorption of sodium or chloride may be abnormal in patients with Bartter's syndrome, resulting in a greater than normal amount of filtered sodium being delivered to the distal nephron, where it is exchanged for potassium or excreted in the urine. The unusual combination of elevated plasma, angiotensin II, and aldosterone levels and a normal blood pressure suggested that the disorder might be accompanied by synthesis of abnormally large amounts of a vasodepressor substance. Subsequently, Gill et al.[250] have demonstrated that patients with Bartter's syndrome excrete a large amount of PGE$_2$, and Halushka et al.[251] have found increased urinary kallikrein excretion. Since indomethacin prevents the synthesis of all of the products of the cyclooxygenase reaction, including PGE$_2$, this agent was used to treat patients with Bartter's syndrome[252] and was found to be remarkably effective in reversing the characteristic pathophysiologic disorders of this syndrome. In these patients, the administration of indomethacin partially corrected the elevated plasma renin, angiotensin, and aldosterone levels; the renal loss of salt and water was reduced, and the pressor responsiveness to angiotensin and norepinephrine was restored.[250, 251]

It is attractive to attribute all of these effects to the inhibition of one or more products of the cyclooxygenase reaction. However, as noted previously, indomethacin and all other aspirin-like drugs have a variety of actions that might account for some of these effects. The multiplicity of effects of nonsteroidal anti-inflammatory agents on arachidonic acid metabolism in the kidney must also be recognized. The first step in prostaglandin-synthesis is the release of arachidonic acid by the action of an acylhydrolase, phospholipase A$_2$ (see Fig 5–9). The second is the cyclooxygenase step that leads to production of the cyclic endoperoxides. This step is inhibited by indomethacin and similar compounds. Downstream from the generation of endoperoxides is the formation of a number of vasoactive products in different cellular elements within the kidney. Within the vascular wall, stimulation of cyclooxygenase results primarily in the production of PGI_2, a compound that prevents aggregation of platelets and causes vasodilatation.[239] Within the interstitial cells of the renal medulla, stimulation of the cyclooxygenase step results primarily in the production of PGE_2.[253] Within the collecting tubules, prostaglandin synthesis becomes intimately involved with the kallikrein-kinin system and with antidiuretic hormone. Further, these are products of the prostaglandin endoperoxides which require special conditions for their synthesis. Thus, thromboxane A_2, a potent vasoconstrictor, is synthesized in negligible quantities by the normal kidney. However, renal injury, such as ureteral ligation, results in the synthesis of large amounts of thromboxane within the kidney.

It has been proposed that a deficiency in renal prostaglandin production is involved in the pathogenesis of essential hypertension. Campbell et al.[254] have investigated normotensive and hypertensive black and white women and found that sodium depletion increased urinary $PGF_{2\alpha}$ and thromboxane B_2 production in normotensive subjects but not in hypertensive patients. Race and renin status also influenced prostaglandin $F_{2\alpha}$ excretion. The increase in urinary $PGF_{2\alpha}$ excretion was seen only in black and normal-renin hypertensive patients and not in white or low-renin hypertensive patients. With sodium loading, there were no consistent changes in excretion of any of the three compounds measured; however, urinary kallikrein excretion did rise with sodium intake. Thus, the only difference between hypertensive and normotensive subjects was an attenuation in the increase in excretion of prostaglandins that was ordinarily seen during sodium depletion.

Lebel and Grose[255] examined urinary excretion of PGE_2 and $PGF_{2\alpha}$ in normal and hypertensive subjects and found that 12% of the hypertensive patients had extremely low levels of urinary PGE_2, but the average values for the normal and hypertensive patients was not significantly different. There was no relationship between urinary prostaglandins in the level of blood pressure, plasma renin activity, or sodium excretion.

Ruilope et al.[256] studied urinary PGE_2 excretion in normal subjects and hypertensive patients and found elevated PGE_2 excretion in normal renin essential hypertension, while low-renin essential hypertensive patients excreted values that were lower than those of normal subjects. In this study, plasma renin activity and urinary PGE_2 excretion were found to be significantly related. Indomethacin reduced excretion of PGE_2 in normal subjects and normal-renin hypertensive subjects but not in low-renin essential hypertensives. In addition, indomethacin resulted in further increases in blood pressure in normal-renin essential hypertensive patients.

Sato et al.[257] studied the effect of dietary sodium intake on the renal metabolism of prostaglandins and found that a low-sodium intake increased urinary excretion of the main metabolites of $PGF_{2\alpha}$ but not of prostaglandin E_2 or $F_{2\alpha}$ itself. A high-sodium intake increased the urinary excretion of PGE_2. Increasing dietary intake of potassium did not affect urinary excretion of prostaglandins.

Rathaus and Bernheim[258] studied the effect of propranolol on urinary excretion of prostaglandins E_2 and $F_{2\alpha}$ in normal subjects and patients with essential hypertension. They found that urinary excretion of PGE_2 increased significantly after propranolol, while that of $PGF_{2\alpha}$ did not change. After furosemide was given intravenously, treatment with propranolol increased PGE_2 response. Prostaglandin $F_{2\alpha}$ increased in response to furosemide before propranolol treatment, but after β-blockade, there was no effect.

Interrelationships of Prostaglandins and the Kallikrein-Kinin System

Bradykinin is a potent vasodilator peptide. When infused into the renal artery, it causes natriuresis and diuresis[259, 260] which might be secondary to changes in renal blood flow. Two separate systems exist in man for the formation of kinins.[261] In plasma, prekallikrein, which is synthesized in the liver,[262] is acted upon by prekallikrein activators to form active kallikrein. This proteolytic enzyme, in turn, acts on plasma kininogens to generate bradykinin. The active peptide is lysed by kininases in plasma and tissues.

The cells of the distal renal tubule synthesize urinary kallikrein.[263, 264] In the distal segments of the nephron, this enzyme acts on kininogen to generate lysyl-bradykinin,[263] which in turn is cleaved by an aminopeptidase to form bradykinin.[261] While little of the bradykinin that is infused into the renal artery or proximal tubules is recovered in the urine,[265, 266] bradykinin that is infused into the distal tubule is almost completely recovered.

Although the physiologic role of the kallikrein-kinin system remains incompletely understood, two facts appear to be well established. First, sodium-retaining hormones increase urinary kallikrein excretion; this can be interpreted as evidence to support the hypothesis that kinins have a primary role in the regulation of salt and water balance, or alternatively, a secondary response.[267, 268] Second, interventions that alter extracellular fluid volume affect plasma renin activity and plasma bradykinin levels similarly.[268, 269, 270, 271] A rise in bradykinin levels at a time when angiotensin II levels are high might serve to protect against excessive vasoconstriction during salt depletion or volume loss. It can be further proposed that either excess activity of pressor elements in this balance or inadequate activity of vasodepressor elements can result in hypertension. Prostaglandins interact with both elements, reinforcing the activity of the kallikrein-kinin system and blunting the influence of the renin-angiotensin system.[272]

Kinins can be involved in the action of prostaglandins in several ways (Fig 5–11). Bradykinin activates a phospholipase[273] that releases arachidonic acid and increases synthesis of prostaglandins.[274] Kinins also stimulate PGE-9-ketoreductase,[275] which results in the conversion of PGE_2 to $PGF_{2\alpha}$.[168] These two actions may explain the venoconstrictor effect of the kinins.

Prostaglandins and kinins may also interact locally, within the tissue in which they are formed. The vasodilation evoked by bradykinin in

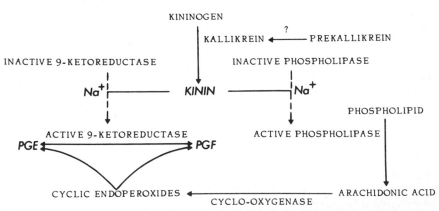

Fig 5–11.—Kinin-prostaglandin interactions. Kinin increases prostaglandin synthesis by making more substrate available to the synthase complex. Kinins also may regulate production of the major end-product, a PGE or PGF, by activating the enzyme, PGE-9-ketoreductase. Activation of 9-ketoreductase is possibly sensitive to either sodium or other ions. (From the Federation of American Society for Experimental Biology, taken from McGiff J.C., et al.: Modulation and mediation of the action of the renal kallikreinkinin system by prostaglandins. *Fed. Proc.* 35:175, 1976. Used by permission.)

vascular tissue is an example of modulation of the action of kinins by prostaglandins,[276] whereas the venoconstrictor effect of the kinins in mesenteric veins[168] and the actions of the kinins on the urine concentration[277] are examples of prostaglandin release mediating the effects of kinins. Finally, the level of activity of the kallikrein-kinin system may influence the basal generation of prostaglandins, which contributes to the maintenance of normal blood flow in the kidney[278, 169] and gravid uterus.[279]

Interrelationships of the Renin-Angiotensin and Kallikrein-Kinin Systems

There are many similarities between the two systems (Fig 5–12). Both renin and kallikrein are proteolytic enzymes that are formed and stored within the kidney, both may be released by the autonomic nervous system, and both act on plasma globulins to release decapeptides, angiotensin I, and lysyl-bradykinin. Each decapeptide is converted to an octapeptide by angiotensin-converting enzyme or kininase II,[280] which profoundly affects its activity; angiotensin I undergoes conversion to angiotensin II while bradykinin undergoes degradation.[281] Both bradykinin and angiotensin II release prostaglandins from several tissues; infusion of either one causes renal venous prostaglandin concentrations to rise 10%–50% above control levels.[228, 282] The effector compounds in the two systems, angiotensin II and bradykinin, have opposite pressor effects, which may serve to balance one another. Several clinical studies have demonstrated parallel increases in the activity of the renin-angiotensin and kallikrein-kinin systems[268, 269, 271] in response to stimuli that alter effective intravascular volume, such as salt depletion and upright posture. For example, enhanced activity of the kallikrein-kinin system may, in part, explain the absence of hypertension in patients with Bartter's syndrome.[251]

The Kallikrein-Kinin System in Human Hypertension

Urinary excretion of kallikrein is decreased in human and experimental forms of hypertension.[283, 284] A radiochemical assay for urinary

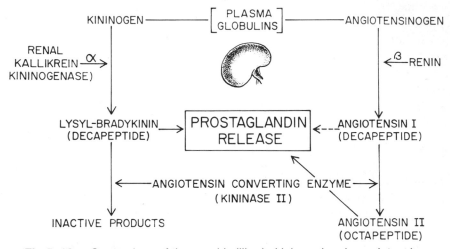

Fig 5–12.—Comparison of the renal kallikrein-kinin and renin-angiotensin systems. The symbols α and β above the arrows proceeding from kallikrein and kinin, respectively, refer to adrenergic mechanisms which participate in the regulation of kallikrein (α) and renin (β) release.
　　The major products of each system are capable of releasing prostaglandins. Angiotensin-converting enzyme, which increases the activity of the renin-angiotensin system by conversion of angiotensin I to the more active form, angiotensin II, correspondingly reduces the activity of the kallikrein-kinin system by degrading lysyl-bradykinin to inactivative products. (From the Federation of American Society for Experimental Biology, taken from McGiff J.C., et al.: Modulation and mediation of the action of the renal kallikreinkinin system by prostaglandins. *Fed. Proc.* 35:175, 1976. Used by permission.)

kallikrein[285] has made it possible to study large populations of hypertensive subjects and their families.[286, 287] Although changes in kallikrein excretion are assumed to reflect changes in the activity of the kallikrein-kinin system intrarenally, this does not take into account the importance of kininases as regulators of the levels of kinins, nor does it take into account alterations in the amounts of substrate made available at sites in the kidney. Renal kininase activity is ordinarily high.[265] Reduced activity can result in increases in the levels of kinins within the kidney. Nasjletti et al.[265, 288] have shown that inhibition of kininase II by the nonapeptide $BPP_{9\alpha}$ increased renal blood flow and sodium excretion. These changes reflect increased intrarenal generation of endogenous kinins and were associated with increased levels of kinins in urine and renal venous blood. An increase of kallikrein excretion is not essential for a change in intrarenal levels of kinins to occur.

Many subjects with essential hypertension excrete less kallikrein than do normotensive subjects, and they have decreased responsiveness to stimuli that increase kallikrein excretion.[267] The lower secretory rates are found in the hypertensive black subject, although the normotensive black subject shows decreased kallikrein excretion when compared to normal white subjects matched for age and sex.[286] These differences were not related to variations in urinary sodium and potassium excretion or volume.

An examination of the relationships among urinary kallikrein, plasma renin activity, and renal blood flow suggests that a vasodilator system, the kallikrein-kinin-prostaglandin, participates in the regulation of vascular resistance in the kidney, together with the renin-angiotensin system. In the dog with renal arterial stenosis, decreased kallikrein excretion correlates with renal blood flow, not with changes in either urinary volume or sodium excretion.[289] Both vasoconstrictor and vasodilator agents can release renal kallikrein. The signal for kallikrein release is probably a change in transmural pressure, since blunting of kallikrein release has been reported after renal compliance was reduced by wrapping the kidney with latex.[290] A study of hypertensive patients with unilateral renal arterial stenosis provided additional evidence that the kallikrein-kinin system is less active in the ischemic kidney and that the activities of the renin-angiotensin and kallikrein-kinin systems are inversely related.[291] In this study, plasma renin activity was elevated and kinin levels were depressed in the venous effluent of the diseased kidney, whereas the reverse obtained for the contralateral kidney.

Studies of kallikrein excretion in hypertension have made important contributions to our understanding of the pathogenesis and inheritance of hypertension.[292] Decreased concentration of urinary kallikrein has been shown in both black children and black adults. Since these children were not clinically hypertensive, a relationship was sought between urinary kallikrein and the level of blood pressure within these families. Both diastolic and systolic blood pressures in the families with the lowest urinary kallikrein concentrations were significantly higher than in those families showing the highest urinary kallikrein concentrations. Measurements that were repeated three years later in the same population confirmed the original results.[287] These studies support the hypothesis that a deficiency of the kallikrein-kinin system contributes to the development of high blood pressure in a susceptible population.

O'Connor[293] has studied urinary kallikrein activity in patients with essential hypertension treated with propranolol and found that this β-blocking agent diminished urinary kallikrein excretion at the same time that renal blood flow and blood pressure were reduced. However, the change in renal blood flow did not correlate with the change in kallikrein excretion. O'Connor and his co-workers[294] have also studied urinary kallikrein excretion after renal transplantation and found that urinary kallikrein appeared to originate in the transplanted kidney. Urinary excretion of kallikrein was lower in the hypertensive recipients of transplants than in normotensive subjects. Patients who developed acute tubular necrosis or kidney rejection also excreted less kallikrein than those who did not.

Saruta and Kondo[295] have studied urinary kallikrein excretion and other endocrine factors in young patients with essential hypertension. Most of these individuals had a normal plasma renin activity. However, when subjects were grouped into low- (10.7%), normal- (55.4%), and high- (33.9%) renin groups, it was noted that urinary excretion of kallikrein was increased in the high-renin group and reduced in the low-renin group.

The major exception to the conclusion that hypertension is usually associated with deficient kallikrein excretion is mineralocorticoid-induced hypertension;[296] aldosteronism is associated with increased excretion of kallikrein. Kallikrein excretion is also elevated in normotensive subjects when mineralocorticoid activity is augmented by administration of sodium-retaining steroids or by sodium restriction. It was demonstrated that kallikrein excretion that is elevated by a low-sodium diet can be decreased by spironolactone; this led to the proposal that the concentration of mineralocorticoids determines the rate of kallikrein excretion.[296] An alternative explanation is that a consequence of elevated mineralocorticoid activity, such as increased potassium excretion, may play a decisive role in increasing kallikrein-kinin activity. Urinary kallikrein concentration has been positively correlated with potassium excretion[292] but not with sodium excretion. Decreased extracellular potassium, resulting from increased excretion, may result in enhanced renal prostaglandin synthesis, which may augment the activity of the renal kallikrein-kinin system. Changes in extracellular potassium concentration can affect renal prostaglandin synthesis,[297, 253] which in turn affects kallikrein release and/or kinin generation, perhaps by operating through a kallikrein-releasing mechanism similar to the prostaglandin mechanism that regulates renin release.[298]

The intrarenal kinin levels may be of greater importance than kallikrein excretion. Vinci et al.[299] have shown that over a wide range of excretion of kallikrein, urinary kinin levels were not affected. They also noted that urinary excretion of kinins was independent of the level of mineralocorticoids in normal subjects.

The relationship between sodium excretion and the activity of the renal kallikrein-kinin system is uncertain. In most of the studies that addressed the effects of altered activity of the renal kallikrein-kinin system on salt and water excretion, the changes in kallikrein excretion were measured rather than the changes in kinin levels. However, Marin-Grez et al.[300] measured changes in urinary kallikrein excretion and kinin levels in the caval blood of the dog in response to acute expansion of extracellular fluid volume induced by sodium. They found a positive correlation between changes in blood levels of kinins of renal origin and changes in sodium excretion induced by saline administration. Three studies suggest that the renal kallikrein-kinin system, perhaps in concert with renal prostaglandins, participates in regulating sodium chloride excretion: First, Nasjletti et al.[301] have demonstrated a relationship between the transient decrease in urinary sodium in the conscious rat produced by the kallikrein inhibitor, aprotinin, and the immediate reduction in PGE excretion. Second, in the dog, enhancement of the activity of the renal kallikrein-kinin system by inhibition of the degradative enzyme, kininase II, was associated with natriuresis.[265] Third, in the rat, antibodies of bradykinin have been shown to attenuate the enhanced excretion of sodium chloride in response to acute isotonic saline loading.[302]

Since changes in kinin generation have profound effects on prostaglandin levels within the kidney,[303] and since prostaglandins may contribute to the effects of kinins on salt and water excretion,[277] prostaglandins should be measured simultaneously with the components of the kallikrein-kinin system in order to assess the effects of changes in either on salt and water excretion. In view of the wide distribution of prostaglandin-synthesizing enzymes among the cellular elements of the kidney,[240] it is important to recognize that compartmentalization of kinin and prostaglandin metabolism may have important consequences for renal function (Fig 5–13). The functional result of the interactions of the renal kallikrein-kinin and prostaglandin systems may be restricted to the urinary compartment. Entry of kallikrein into the distal tubules[304] and subsequent formation of kinin, then, may result in kinin-mediated generation of prostaglandins in the distal nephron and collecting ducts; the latter affects the excretion of free water.[277] A study by Weber et al.[305] indicates that a major prostaglandin-metabolizing enzyme, PGE_2-9-ketoreductase, which converts PGE_2 to $PGF_{2\alpha}$, is influenced by sodium balance. Thus, the retention of a water load and the conservation of sodium is facilitated by the increased activity of this enzyme, which lowers levels of PGE_2 intrarenally by favoring formation of $PGF_{2\alpha}$. As prostaglandins of the E series inhibit ADH activity,[170]

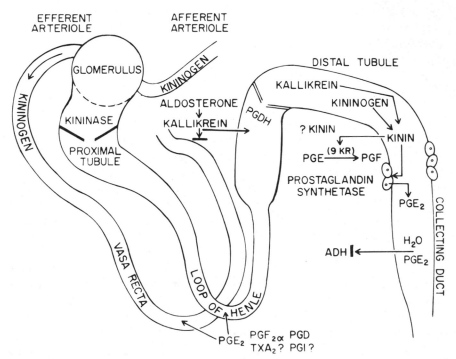

Fig 5–13.—Prostaglandin-kinin interaction in the nephron. The generation of kinins in the distal nephron and collecting ducts releases prostaglandins which inhibit the effect of ADH and, thereby, participate in the excretion of solute free water: Prostaglandin 15-hydroxy-dehydrogenase *(PGDH)*, PGE-9-ketoreductase *(9KR)*. (From the Federation of American Society for Experimental Biology, taken from McGiff J.C., et al.: Modulation and mediation of the action of the renal kallikrein-kinin system by prostaglandins. *Fed. Proc.* 35:17, 1976. Used by permission.)

their conversion of PGF facilitates reabsorption of water. Kinins can also influence PGE_2-9-ketoreductase activity.[275] This interaction may explain the effects of kinins on free-water generation. When prostaglandins are released through the actions of kinins, free water is generated if PGE_2 is the principal product, whereas when $PGF_{2\alpha}$ is released in response to kinin, water conservation occurs. The activity of PGE_2-9-ketoreductase, modified by kinins, may be a function of the state of sodium chloride balance. It is here that a hypertensive mechanism may be provoked; deficient intrarenal generation of kinins or prostaglandins in response to salt intake may result in inappropriate expansion of extracellular fluid volume, a recognized factor in the pathogenesis of hypertension.[59]

Although the physiologic role of the kallikrein-kinin system in the kidney has not been proved, it appears to be related to renovascular dilatation and natriuresis. Both kallikrein and kinin are excreted in the urine but not always in relation to each other. The excretion of kallikrein is influenced by changes in the activity of the renin-angiotensin-aldosterone system as well as by changes in diet. Hypertension, particularly renal parenchymal hypertension, appears to reduce kallikrein excretion. Kallikrein excretion rises when dietary sodium is restricted. Similarly, kallikrein excretion rises when thiazide diuretics are administered.[306] O'Connor[306] found that individuals who respond to thiazides have a greater increase in urinary kallikrein excretion than those who fail to respond, which suggests that the renal kallikreins may be involved in the antihypertensive effects of thiazide diuretics.

In summary, the main effects of prostaglandins involve local regulation rather than an endocrine function. Prostaglandins synthesized in the vasculature promote vasodilation, while those synthesized locally in the kidney affect vasodilation and natriuresis. The synthesis of prostaglandins by the kidney is stimulated by circumstances that interfere with renal perfusion, e.g., vasoconstriction or hypotension. Interactions of prostaglandins, the renin-angiotensin system, the kallikrein-kinin system, the sympathetic nervous system, circulatory regulatory centers in the central nervous system, vascular endothelium and smooth muscle, and renal tubular epithelial cells control blood pressure by direct and indirect effects on the heart and blood vessels and on renal excretion of sodium and water.

VASODEPRESSOR LIPIDS

Recent research suggests that the kidney influences blood pressure in yet another way, through the release of vasodepressor lipids. Muirhead et al.[307] have shown that both renal medullary tissues and interstitial cells from the renal medulla that are grown in tissue culture elaborate lipid compounds, which, when infused into experimental animals, reduce arterial pressure. It has been shown that transplanted renal medullary tissue from normotensive animals protects against the development of both renoprival, one-kidney, one-clip sodium-overload hypertension and genetic hypertension.[308] However, transplants of renal cortical tissue or tissues from organs other than the kidney do not have the same protective effect. Renal interstitial cells that have been grown in tissue culture and transplanted were found also to protect against the development of hypertension.[309] Tobian and Azar,[310] Manthorpe,[311] and Susic et al.[312] have confirmed this antihypertensive function of the kidney. Gothberg et al.[313] have published data suggesting that the release of vasodepressor lipids is responsible for rapid fall in blood pressure after removal of the clip in rats with two-kidney, one-clip hypertension.

Muirhead and his co-workers[314] have distinguished two types of antihypertensive medullary lipids based on their differences in solubility and chromatographic behavior. One lipid is a highly polar glycerophospholipid that has been designated "antihypertensive polar renal medullary lipid." The other compound, "antihypertensive neutral medullary lipid," differs from the polar lipid in that it does not require chemical reduction to become biologically active. Both compounds, given intravenously, lower blood pressure. The antihypertensive polar renal medullary lipid has been given intravenously to hypertensive rats and found to reduce blood pressure by lowering peripheral vascular resistance. The antihypertensive neutral renal medullary lipid lowers blood pressure while at the same time reducing heart rate and increasing efferent renal nerve activity, which suggests that a central nervous system action is involved in the antihypertensive effect of this compound. Faber et al.[315] have recently studied the regional hemodynamic effects of both antihypertensive renal medullary lipids in conscious rats. The compounds were infused both intravenously and into the central nervous system of rats with and without sino-aortic deafferentation. The results suggested that neither lipid had an effect mediated through the central nervous system. Nonetheless, both lipids were again shown to be potent vasodepressor agents. The antihypertensive polar renal medullary lipid was found to have strong peripheral vasodilatory effects, and it also reduced the response to vasoconstrictor agents.

These observations have led Muirhead to propose that a deficiency in elaboration of antihypertensive radiomedullary lipids plays a role, perhaps a permissive one, in the development of hypertension.[316]

MEMBRANE TRANSPORT AND HYPERTENSION

Considerable evidence has been accumulated in recent years that suggests that the genetic predisposition to hypertension noted in human beings might be due to abnormalities of electrolyte transport across various cell membranes. In 1975, Edmundson[317] reported that the rate of extrusion of sodium from the white blood cells of patients with essential hypertension was impaired, resulting in an increased concentration of sodium within the white cell. Subsequently, a number of studies have been carried out demonstrating that there are at least three systems of sodium transport in the wall of certain human cells. These investigations have usually used red blood cells because of their easy availability. One transport system is an energy-requiring sodium-potassium pump, which requires lysis of adenosine triphosphate for activity. This system is inhibited by ouabain and by endoxin, a digoxin-like substance that appears in the circulation of animals and man subjected to volume overload. A second system is the sodium-potassium cotransport that results in a coupled transmembrane efflux or influx of sodium and potassium. Third, a lithium-sodium exchange or countertransport system exchanges sodium or lithium for sodium across the plasma membrane. The latter two systems are not inhibited by ouabain; however, the sodium-potassium cotransport system is inhibited by furosemide.

Garay and his colleagues[318] have studied sodium-potassium cotransport in normal subjects, subjects with essential hypertension, and those with secondary hypertension, and they found that outward cotransport of both sodium and potassium was reduced in the red blood cells of most patients with essential hypertension and in the normotensive offspring of hypertensive parents. Patients with secondary forms of hypertension were not found to have impaired cotransport. These observations have stimulated considerable research into possible abnormalities of the sodium-potassium cotransport system in various populations; this research has produced conflicting results. Three studies[319, 320] have found impaired sodium-potassium cotransport, whereas three others[321, 322, 323] have not confirmed the presence of an abnormality. However, considerable differences in methodology were used in the various studies.

Adragna et al.[324] demonstrated elevated erythrocyte sodium-potassium cotransport in white subjects with essential hypertension, whereas Tuck et al.[325] have demonstrated low cotransport in black normotensive subjects.

Ghione et al.[319] and Cusi et al.[320] have demonstrated impaired sodium-potassium cotransport in the red blood cells of patients with essential hypertension. In contrast, Swarts et al.,[321] Walter and Distler,[322] and Duhm et al.[323] have failed to show an abnormality of cotransport in patients with essential hypertension.

Canessa et al.[326] studied sodium-lithium countertransport in the red blood cells of patients with essential hypertension, and they found that increased activity characterizes this particular sodium transport system in the hypertensive subject. The countertransport system was also found to be abnormal in normotensive first-degree relatives of the subjects with essential hypertension. Most other studies of sodium-lithium transport, by Woods et al.,[327] Travisan et al.,[328] and Brugnara et al.[329] have also shown an abnormality of countertransport in the erythrocytes of subjects with essential hypertension. However, Duhm and Gobel[330] and Isben et al.[331] using modified methods, failed to confirm the presence of abnormal sodium-lithium countertransport in hypertensive patients.

Thus, the weight of evidence points to abnormalities of sodium transport in the cell membranes of hypertensive subjects, although the exact nature and distribution of this abnormality awaits additional research and further standardization of techniques. The present data

TABLE 5–2.—CARDIOVASCULAR, RENAL AND ENDOCRINE CHANGES DURING HYPERTENSION AND PREGNANCY

	UNCOMPLICATED ESSENTIAL HYPERTENSION	NORMAL PREGNANCY	PREGNANCY-INDUCED HYPERTENSION
Cardiovascular			
Arterial Pressure	Increased	Reduced	Increased
Cardiac Output	Normal or Increased	Increased	Increased
Systemic Vascular Resistance	Increased	Decreased	Increased
Vascular Reactivity	Increased	Decreased	Increased
Uterine Blood Flow		Increased	Reduced
Renal			
Renal Blood Flow	Increased Early Decreases with Severity	Increased	Decreased
Glomerular Filtration Rate	Unchanged	Increased	Decreased
Plasma Volume	Contracted	Expanded	Contracted
Total Body Sodium	Normal	Increased	Increased
Intracellular Sodium	Increased	Decreased in 2nd Trimester	Normal
Endocrine			
Plasma Catecholamines	Normal to Increased	Unchanged	Unchanged
Plasma Renin Activity	High, Low, or Normal	Increased	Decreased
Plasma Aldosterone	Normal	Increased	Decreased
Plasma PGE_2 and PGI_2	Normal	Increased	Decreased
Urinary Kallikrein	Decreased	Increased	Decreased

suggest that the most reproducible abnormality is that of sodium-lithium countertransport.

Blaustein[81] has postulated that if an abnormality of sodium transport reduces extrusion of sodium from intracellular spaces and accumulates sodium within the intracellular space, this would in turn enhance sodium-calcium exchange across cell membranes, resulting in a net increase of intracellular calcium concentration. In the case of contractile cells, such as the vascular smooth muscle that makes up the resistance arteriole, or the myocardium, this would result in enhanced contractility. A relatively increased cardiac output against a relatively fixed vascular resistance would in turn elevate blood pressure.

COMPARISON OF ESSENTIAL AND PREGNANCY-INDUCED HYPERTENSION

The abnormalities of cardiovascular, renal, and endocrine function that have been described in patients with uncomplicated essential hypertension are summarized in Table 5–2. These changes are contrasted with those reported to occur during normal pregnancy and those observed in patients with pregnancy-induced hypertension. The latter will be described in the following section.

CHAPTER 6

PREGNANCY-INDUCED HYPERTENSION: ETIOLOGIC CONSIDERATIONS

IMMENSE GAPS REMAIN in our understanding of pregnancy-induced hypertension. The etiology or etiologies of preeclampsia-eclampsia, the specific diseases of pregnancy, are not known. Initially it was believed that the gravid uterus released toxic products into the circulation to produce a group of otherwise unrelated diseases gathered under the heading of "the toxemias of pregnancy." With time, it has become clear that some of these conditions are due to other causes. For example, acute yellow atrophy of the liver following hyperemesis gravidarum is associated with deficiency of sulfur-containing amino acids, and Wernicke's encephalopathy is associated with thiamine deficiency. The origin of the term *eclampsia* has been reviewed by Chesley.[332] This word, of Greek origin, refers to a "shining forth" and has been used to describe changes of youth and early adulthood. In 1682, Castelli defined *eclampsia* as "a brightness, lightning, effulgence or shining forth," referring to writings attributed to Hippocrates.[333] The use of this word to describe the sudden appearance of convulsions is attributed to Bossier de Sauvages in 1739. De Sauvages referred to all convulsions of acute etiology as eclampsia and distinguished this condition from epilepsy, which he considered to be a different chronic disease. In later writings he described several types of eclampsia related to hemorrhage, pain, helminthic infection, or other conditions.[334] This use of the word continued for around 200 years. It was not until the 1961 edition of *Sted-*

73

man's Medical Dictionary that nonobstetrical meanings of this term were no longer given, and *eclampsia* was defined as "coma and convulsions that may develop during or immediately after pregnancy, related to proteinuria, edema, and hypertension."[335]

IMPAIRED UTEROPLACENTAL PERFUSION

Over the years, considerable evidence has been gathered demonstrating reduced uteroplacental perfusion in hypertensive gravidas compared to those with a normal pregnancy. Gant et al.[336] have presented evidence that the metabolic clearance of dehydroisoandrosterone sulfate is related to uteroplacental blood flow and have used this technique to demonstrate reduced flow in patients with preeclampsia (Fig 6–1). The most recent study in this area is that of Lunnell et al.,[337] who used intravenously administered indium 113 and a computer-linked probe to measure uteroplacental blood flow in 32 patients with preeclampsia and 37 normal control subjects. Uteroplacental flow was measured as an index calculated from the ascending limb and the maximum activity of the isotope accumulation curve. A 50% reduction of uteroplacental perfusion was found in the patients with preeclampsia. The most severely affected patients had the greatest impairment of flow. A reduction of flow was found even in those patients with no evidence of intrauterine growth retardation. Of note was the observation that rest in the supine position reduced uteroplacental flow by one third compared to flow measured in the left lateral decubitus position. A possible explanation is provided by the observations of Sullivan, Prewitt, and Josephs, who found attenuation of the conjunctival microvasculature in young subjects with early borderline hypertension[56] (Figs 6–2, 6–3). If these changes involve the uterine circulation, it might not be possible for a hypertensive gravida to have uterine blood flow increase during pregnancy to the same degree as a normotensive woman.

Because hypertensive pregnancies are associated with reduced uteroplacental blood flow, it has been postulated that impaired uteroplacental circulation is the underlying cause of preeclampsia. Page[338] proposed that impaired placental circulation is followed by the development of pathologic changes in the placenta, the escape of tro-

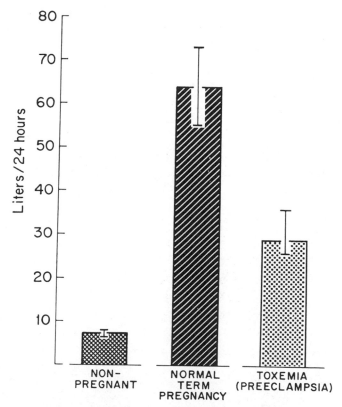

Fig 6–1.—Metabolic clearance rate of dehydroisoandrosterone sulfate (DS). The values for the nonpregnant groups were obtained from 2 normal men and 2 normal young women. The mean value for metabolic clearance of DS in the normal term pregnant subjects was derived from 15 measurements in both primigravid and multigravid women. Values for metabolic clearance of DS in the preeclamptic group were obtained from 6 primigravid women with hypertension, edema, and proteinuria. (From Gant N.F., et al.: Study of the metabolic clearance rate of dehydroisoandrosterone sulfate in pregnancy. *Am. J. Obstet. Gynecol.* 111:555–563, 1971. Used by permission.)

phoblast, and the subsequent development of slow, disseminated intravascular coagulation as depicted in Figure 6–4. Products of coagulation which are formed within the circulation are later deposited within the glomeruli, possibly producing the glomerular endothelial lesions that characterize preeclampsia. These lesions are accompanied by a reduced glomerular filtration rate and sodium retention. Subsequent intracellular shifts of sodium cause edema and increased arteriolar re-

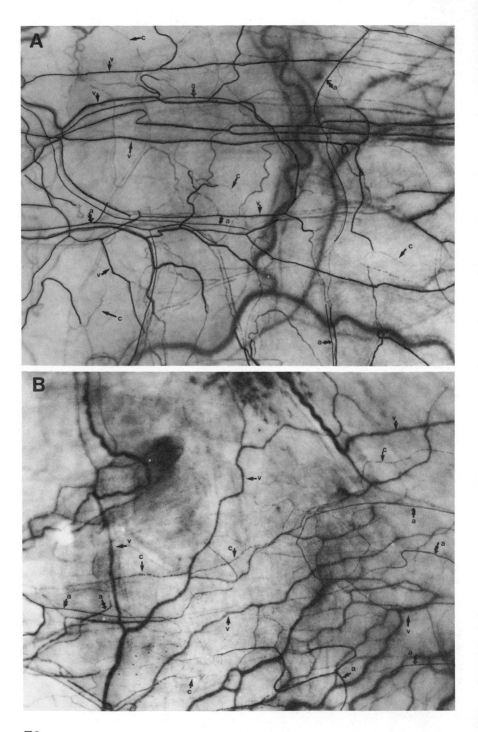

76

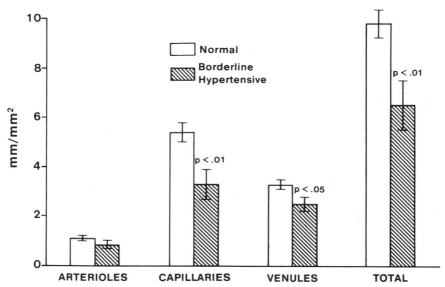

Fig 6–3.—Conjunctival vessel length densities, comparing normal with borderline hypertensive subjects. (From Sullivan J.M., et al.: Attenuation of the microcirculation in young patients with high-output borderline hypertension. *Hypertension* 5:844–851, 1983. Used by permission of the American Heart Association.)

sponsiveness to pressor substances. The latter leads to vasoconstriction which further reduces uteroplacental circulation and perpetuates the cycle, leading to impaired renal function, rapid disseminated intravascular coagulation, and the seizures that characterize eclampsia.

In experimental animals, the injection of serotonin causes lesions resembling those of preeclampsia. In normal pregnant subjects, plasma serotonin levels increase, but they do not increase further in preeclampsia, although placental serotonin levels have been reported to increase.[339] This has been attributed to ischemic placental injury with subsequent loss of monoamide oxidase activity. It has been shown that 5-hydroxytryptamine metabolism is reduced in preeclampsia, while the metabolism of tryptamine is not affected.[340]

Fig 6–2.—Fifty-fold magnification of lateral bulbar conjunctival vessels of a normal subject **(A)** and a patient with borderline hypertension **(B).** Examples of arterioles are indicated by *(a)*, venules by *(v)*, and capillaries by *(c)*. (From Sullivan J.M., et al.: Attenuation of the microcirculation in young patients with high-output borderline hypertension. *Hypertension* 5:844–851, 1983. Used by permission of the American Heart Association.)

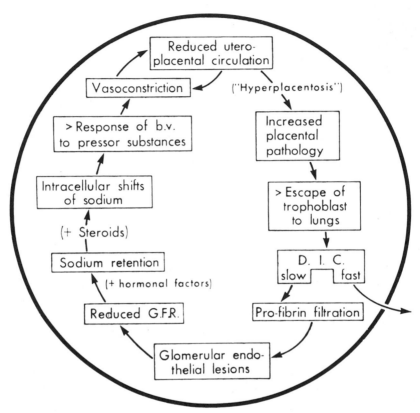

Fig 6–4.—The inner vicious circle of preeclampsia and eclampsia. *D.I.C.*, disseminated intravascular coagulation; *G.F.R.*, glomerular filtration rate. (From Page E.W.: On the pathogenesis of pre-eclampsia and eclampsia. *J. Obstet. Gynaecol. Br. Commonw.* 79:883–894, 1972. Used by permission.)

CARDIOVASCULAR CHANGES IN HYPERTENSIVE PREGNANCY

Cardiovascular function during pregnancy-induced hypertension has been studied and contrasted with the changes seen in normal pregnancy and in pregnancy occurring in patients with essential hypertension. These observations have not uncovered the etiology of pre-eclampsia-eclampsia, but they have produced a number of findings that deserve further study. Hamilton found average cardiac output to be higher in patients with preeclampsia than in patients with normal pregnancies or patients with essential hypertension and pregnancy,[39] but Werko and co-workers found little difference among the three groups in late stages of pregnancy, e.g., 7.3, 7.4, and 7.1 L/min, respectively, during the last 3 weeks of pregnancy.[341] Muscle and liver blood flow has been found to be slightly higher in women with preeclampsia,[342, 343] while cerebral blood flow does not differ.[21, 22] Insulin and para-aminohippuric acid clearance are reduced in preeclampsia,[344] and uterine blood flow has been found to be reduced in pregnant patients with blood pressure elevation.[345] Patients with preeclampsia-eclampsia do not have as great an increase in blood volume as is seen in normal pregnancy.[341, 346] Werko and Brody[347] have found less diurnal variation of blood pressure in patients with preeclampsia than in patients with essential hypertension. Smith et al.[348] have restudied the hemodynamic changes occurring during pregnancy in 10 normal subjects, 16 patients with preeclampsia and 7 patients with essential hypertension and pregnancy. They found cardiac index to be lower in patients with preeclampsia and essential hypertension: 4.5 L/m/sq m in normal subjects versus 3.2 L and 3.3 L in hypertensive subjects. They also found that changes in plasma volume were not as great in patients with the two forms of hypertension. In addition, the uterine-placental turnover rate was lower in both groups with blood pressure elevation.[348]

In more recent studies, Carlsson[349] has shown that preeclampsia was associated with a hyperdynamic circulation characterized by an increased cardiac output, systemic vascular resistance, and arterial blood pressure, despite a contracted plasma volume. He warned that measures taken to expand plasma volume without adequate hemodynamic monitoring could lead to pulmonary and/or cerebral edema because of the hemodynamic characteristics of preeclampsia.

Ku'zniar et al.[350] have used M-mode echocardiography to study hemodynamics in 19 patients with preeclampsia, 9 with essential hypertension, and 19 with normal pregnancies. Although the mean values for heart rate, stroke volume, and cardiac index among the groups did not differ significantly, several significant correlations were found, including an inverse relationship between blood pressure and cardiac index in the preeclamptic patients, a positive relationship between cardiac index and birth weight, and an inverse relationship between systemic vascular resistance and birth weight. Ku'zniar et al.[351] also used echocardiography to study left ventricular systolic function in 42 preeclamptic patients, 23 normotensive, third-trimester gravidas, and 25 nonpregnant patients and found no differences in left ventricular function between normal gravidas and nonpregnant subjects. Seven percent (3 patients) of the preeclamptic group had diminished indices of contractility, and only 1 had clinical signs of congestive heart failure, demonstrating that the cardiac function is well maintained in most but not all patients with preeclampsia, some of whom have preclinical failure.

Phelan and Yurth[352] placed intra-arterial cannulae and Swan-Ganz right heart catheters in 10 severely preeclamptic patients at term and found that the patients had both relatively elevated cardiac index and systemic vascular resistance as a cause of their elevated pressure. Left ventricular function was found to be hyperdynamic, which fell transiently, immediately post partum, leading to a rise in left ventricular filling and central venous pressures. Within an hour after delivery, left ventricular function had returned to its previous hyperdynamic state.

These recent studies suggest that the great majority of patients with preeclampsia have unimpaired left ventricular function during pregnancy. However, a small number have latent or overt left ventricular failure. Thus, if hemodynamic monitoring does not take place at the time of delivery or during attempts to normalize intravascular volume, a careful and frequent search for clinical evidence of the appearance of pulmonary congestion and edema, such as orthopnea, pulmonary rales, and gallop rhythm, must be carried out.

VASCULAR REACTIVITY IN PREECLAMPSIA-ECLAMPSIA

Vascular reactivity during pregnancies with and without hypertension has been the subject of a number of studies. Dieckmann and co-workers found that preeclampsia-eclampsia developed in 31% of patients with a marked blood pressure rise during a cold pressor test, while only 3% of patients with a normal response developed this disorder.[353] However, in subsequent studies, Browne was unable to confirm this observation.[354]

Although the pressor response to epinephrine or norepinephrine infusion does not differ between pregnant and nonpregnant women,[355, 356, 357] infusion of angiotensin II ordinarily results in a re-

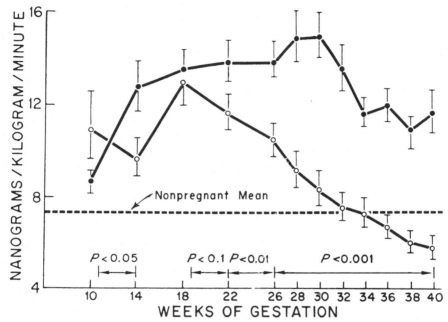

Fig 6–5.—Comparison of mean angiotensin II doses (ng/kg/min) required to evoke a pressor response in 120 primigravidas who remained normotensive and 72 primigravidas who ultimately had pregnancy-induced hypertension. The nonpregnant mean is shown as a broken line. The difference between the two groups became significant after week 23 ($P < .01$). (From Gant N.F., et al.: *J. Clin. Invest.* 52:2682–2689, 1973. Used by permission.)

duced pressor response in normal pregnant subjects[357, 358] (Fig 6–5). This has been attributed to the already high circulating levels of angiotensin II in normal pregnancies,[359, 360] but it also may be a result of increased vascular synthesis of prostaglandins, as discussed in an earlier section. The resistance of angiotensin II cannot be duplicated by the administration of either progesterone or estrogen to nonpregnant women, although progesterone administration will duplicate the reduced antidiuresis and antinatriuresis following angiotension II infusion that is seen in normal pregnancy.[361] In patients with preeclampsia, sensitivity to infused angiotensin II is enhanced but only to the levels seen in nonpregnant subjects.[362, 363] This is not a specific finding, however, since increased sensitivity to the pressor effects of catecholamines[355, 356, 357, 364] and vasopressin[365, 366] have also been reported.

Drugs that induce blockade of the sympathetic ganglia have also been used to study vascular reactivity. Normal pregnant subjects and pregnant subjects with essential hypertension appear to be very sensitive to the administration of ganglionic blocking drugs; blood pressure falls far in excess of that seen in nonpregnant subjects.[367] This observation has led to the suggestion that venous stasis in the lower extremities secondary to uterine enlargement necessitates enhanced sympathetic tone of capacitance vessels in pregnant subjects.[368] In subjects with preeclampsia, marked hypotension after ganglionic blockade does not occur, suggesting that the blood pressure elevation is not mediated by the autonomic nervous system.[369]

RENAL CHANGES IN HYPERTENSIVE PREGNANCY

Marked changes in renal function and sodium and water balance take place during pregnancy.[370] Many of these changes are believed to follow alterations in endocrine status during pregnancy and are considered in greater detail in subsequent sections; this portion focuses on changes within the kidneys and urinary tract.

Throughout a normal pregnancy, glomerular filtration rate increases about 50%, with renal plasma and blood flow increasing about 25%, until late pregnancy.[371, 372, 373] The concentrations of serum creatinine and BUN ordinarily fall during the last months of pregnancy,[373] while renal function tests may also show a decrease prior to delivery. This decrease in function has been attributed to the effect of posture.[374] It has been shown that both glomerular filtration rate and urine flow are decreased more in the standing pregnant subject than in the standing nonpregnant subject.[375] Turning from the lateral decubitus position to the supine position reduces urine flow as much as 56% in the pregnant subject, bringing a corresponding drop in sodium excretion.[374, 376] It has been suggested that mechanical compression of the aorta by the gravid uterus contributes to the reduction in renal function in the supine position.[377] This mechanical effect may also contribute to dilatation of the ureters, renal pelvices, and renal calyces, although alterations in endocrine function are involved in these changes as well.[378, 379] Between the third and eighth month of pregnancy, the magnitude of ureteral peristalsis is decreased.[380] Anatomical changes in the urinary tract revert to normal within 6 weeks of delivery in 94% of patients.[378] Posture is also believed to have an effect of circadian rhythms of renal function in pregnant patients. In the lateral decubitus position, pregnant and nonpregnant patients follow the same pattern of urine output and excretion of creatinine and electrolytes. Assumption of the upright position can reverse day to night ratios in pregnant patients.[381]

Although pregnancy is commonly associated with edema, a number of factors acts to increase sodium loss during normal pregnancy. Progesterone secretion and the amount of unbound plasma progesterone increase during pregnancy.[382] Progesterone has been found to antagonize the effect of aldosterone, acting like spironolactone.[383] The glomerular filtration rate increases during pregnancy and would result in rapid sodium and volume depletion if other factors were not called in to play to increase tubular sodium resorption. A "third factor" has been proposed to explain the natriuresis that occurs with volume expansion in the presence of an increase in glomerular filtration rate. Recent studies have uncovered two compounds that might play a role in this respect. The first, endoxin, is a digoxin-like inhibitor of sodium-potassium ATPase that appears in the circulation during sodium and fluid loading and inhibits sodium resorption in the renal tubules, thus promoting sodium loss but also increasing vascular resistance.[80] The second, atrial natriuretic factor, is formed in granules of the left atrial wall, has vasodilator properties, and is released in response to atrial stretch.[77] Although the roles, if any, of these compounds in normal pregnancy is not known, such a mechanism could conceivably play a role in the salt and water retention associated with preeclampsia.

In a recent report, Beyers et al.[384] described studies that used a commercially available radioimmunoassay kit to measure immunoreactive digoxin-like substance in the blood of 36 patients with normal pregnancies, 21 patients with preeclampsia, and their infants. Levels of digoxin-like substance were higher in cord blood than in maternal blood, and they were higher in the blood of infants born to preeclamptic mothers than in the blood of those born to normal mothers. However, no significant difference between normal and preeclamptic mothers were found. Because endogenous digoxin-like substances are a potential cause of increased vascular resistance, these intriguing findings require confirmation and further study.

Ever since the recognition of pregnancy-induced hypertension as a clinical entity, a number of changes of the renal histology of such patients have been described. In 1918, Lohlein[385] proposed that the major lesion of preeclampsia involved the glomerulus. Several later studies, using light microscopy, described a lesion that was mistakenly believed to be specific for preeclampsia-eclampsia: thickening of the glomerular basement membrane. In 1959 Spargo, McCartney, and Winemiller published their observations on toxemic subjects based on percutaneous renal biopsy and electron microscopy.[386] These investigators described changes primarily involving the capillary endothelium, which they called glomerular endotheliosis. The most characteristic aspect of the lesion was an increase in the endothelial cytoplasm with subsequent narrowing of the capillary lumen. Within the endothelial-cell cytoplasm, droplet and cytoplasmic strand formation, vacuolization, and an increased number of particulate structures were observed. Basement-membrane thickening did not appear to be part of the lesion. Subsequent studies have extended these findings. Increased granularity and enlargement of the juxtaglomerular cells were described by Pollak and Nettles.[387] Mesangial cell proliferation and various deposits between the endothelial cell and the basement membrane were reported by Altcheck, Albright, and Somers.[388] Altchek observed that the typical glomerular changes of preeclampsia can occur with minimal clinical symptoms and can also persist through pregnancy despite control of blood pressure and symptoms with medical therapy.[389] These lesions are also found in patients with essential hypertension who developed proteinuria and edema during pregnancy.[389]

A number of functional renal changes have been observed in patients with preeclampsia and eclampsia. The interpretation of these findings is difficult because of the technical problems imposed by currently available techniques for measuring renal function and by the lack of a diagnosis confirmed by renal biopsy in many studies. Despite these limitations, it seems well established that the glomerular filtration rate is lower in patients with preeclampsia than in comparable subjects with a normal pregnancy.[390, 391] Reduction of effective renal plasma flow has also been described in patients with eclampsia.[391, 392] A lower filtration fraction has been reported in patients with preeclampsia by some investigators,[393, 394] but this has not been a universal finding.[391] McCartney and co-workers carefully studied 22 patients who developed hypertension during pregnancy.[390] Each patient underwent renal biopsy and renal-function studies, which allowed calculation of the quantity of free water extracted per unit of glomerular filtration. This value was reduced in patients with nephrosclerosis or glomerulonephritis but strikingly increased in patients with preeclampsia.

Changes in sodium and water metabolism have also been observed during abnormal pregnancies. It is known that larger quantities of sodium are retained in preeclampsia than in normal pregnancy and that water is retained in excess of sodium.[395] The retention of sodium appears to be greatest in the ambulatory patients.[396] Patients with essential hypertension ordinarily respond to a sodium load with an exaggerated natriuresis. Studies in which the state of sodium balance was carefully defined have demonstrated the same phenomenon in pregnant patients with essential hypertension,[391] although earlier studies suggested diminished natriuresis. Patients with preeclampsia that has been proved by renal biopsy and clinical follow-up, have a lower peak rate of sodium excretion after saline infusion than do subjects with essential hypertension.[391]

ENDOCRINE CHANGES IN NORMAL AND HYPERTENSIVE PREGNANCY

The striking cardiovascular and renal changes observed in uncomplicated pregnancy are accompanied by equally important changes in endocrine function. The growing placenta secretes a number of hormonally active substances that exert their own effects and also require readjustment of the rest of the endocrine system as the pregnant woman enters a new physiologic state. Estriol, 17-β-estradiol, and estrone are normally secreted by the placenta in progressively greater amounts.[397, 398] Estradiol has been demonstrated to cause sodium retention under certain circumstances.[399] The administration of estrogens also increases hepatic production of a number of proteins, including renin substrate.[400, 401] Placental progesterone secretion also increases gradually during pregnancy, reaching a peak at about the 35th week, at which time the progesterone produced is roughly tenfold greater than that produced by the ovaries during the luteal phase of the menstrual cycle.[382] Plasma levels of unbound progesterone are also increased.[382] During the last week of pregnancy, progesterone secretion has been reported to fall slightly.[402] Progesterone is known to cause natriuresis in the presence of aldosterone by antagonizing the sodium-retaining effects of this mineralocorticoid.[383] It has been proposed that the small increase in sodium retention seen in normal pregnant women in the last week of pregnancy is due to a late-gestation fall in progesterone secretion.[402]

A slight increase in plasma and urinary adrenocorticosteroids in late pregnancy also has been reported.[403, 405, 406, 407, 408] Elevated plasma levels of the steroid-binding protein, transcortin, are believed by some to be responsible for the elevation of plasma corticosteroids, although an elevation of free plasma cortisol has also been reported.[409] This provides another possible explanation for the salt retention seen in late pregnancy, since cortisol promotes retention of sodium and excretion of potassium at the distal renal tubule. Studies have shown that free and bound plasma cortisol does not differ in preeclampsia and in normal pregnancy.[410] Data relating to increased pituitary ACTH release during pregnancy are conflicting,[411, 412] although there does appear to be an increase in melanocyte-stimulating hormone.[413] The increase in plasma protein-bound iodine in normal pregnancy appear to be related to increased plasma levels of thyroid-binding protein rather than to increased pituitary secretion of thyroid-stimulating hormone.[414]

During pregnancy the placenta also secretes large amounts of chorionic gonadotropin in the first trimester and smaller but constant amounts during the second and third trimesters.[415] Growth hormone-prolactin is also secreted by the placenta in increasing amounts during pregnancy.[416]

Because of the importance of the renin-angiotensin-aldosterone axis in the regulation of pressure-volume homeostasis in normal subjects and subjects with hypertension, a large number of studies have focused on this topic as it relates to hypertensive pregnancies.[417, 418, 419] Changes in the renin-angiotensin-aldosterone axis take place in patients with normal pregnancy, in patients receiving oral contraceptive agents, and in patients who develop elevated blood pressure with either circumstance. A number of investigators have studied these factors in normal pregnancy and have reported qualitatively varying results.[420, 421, 422, 423, 424, 425, 426] There is general agreement that renin substrate concentration, renin activity, and aldosterone levels all rise during normal pregnancy. During the first trimester, renin concentration is also elevated.[423, 426, 427] Although chorionic tissue produces large amounts of renin that is released into the amniotic fluid, the relation of this source to plasma renin activity during pregnancy is not clear.[428] As mentioned previously, vascular reactivity to angiotensin II, but not to norepinephrine, appears to decrease during normal pregnancy.[357, 358]

The estrogens contained in oral contraceptive agents cause similar changes in the renin-angiotensin-aldosterone axis.[429] In both conditions, hepatic synthesis of renin substrate is increased. This results in high levels of plasma renin activity, plasma angiotensin II concentration, and aldosterone secretion. Plasma renin concentration either rises to a lesser extent or actually falls. Unfortunately, the same changes take place in subjects who develop hypertension and in those who do not develop hypertension, which leaves the etiology of blood pressure elevation unclear.[430] Certain differences between the two groups have recently been reported. Acute volume depletion fails to increase plasma renin activity to expected levels in some patients who develop hypertension on oral contraceptive agents.[431] Another case report describes a patient with contraceptive-induced hypertension whose aldosterone secretion did not suppress normally with salt loading.[432]

Aldosterone secretion has been shown to increase during the course of a normal pregnancy.[433, 434] This elevation appears to be in response to an altered physiologic state and remains responsive to a number of interventions. The administration of salt-retaining mineralocorticoids to pregnant subjects results in sodium retention and reduced aldosterone secretion.[435, 436] Aldosterone secretion and excretion respond appropriately to alterations in dietary sodium intake in pregnancy subjects.[434, 437] Diuretic-induced volume depletion and upright posture both serve to increase aldosterone secretion in normal pregnant subjects.[438, 439] Inhibition of aldosterone secretion with heparin-like compounds in normal pregnant women results in negative sodium balance, which reverses during recovery from the drug effect as aldosterone excretion rises to the high level that is normal for pregnancy.[440] It is reasonable to conclude that aldosterone secretion rises during normal pregnancy in response to a tendency towards sodium and volume depletion; this tendency is secondary to either elevated secretion to progesterone or to the elevation of glomerular filtration rate that occurs during a normal pregnancy.

Because preeclampsia is characterized by excess sodium retention, many studies have attempted to find evidence of abnormal mineralocorticoid activity in patients with these disorders. The cause of the sodium retention remains unknown. An early study demonstrated increased renal excretion of a salt-retaining factor in preeclamptic subjects.[441] When aldosterone could be measured, it was found that patients with preeclampsia excreted less aldosterone than did subjects with a normal pregnancy.[442, 443] Preeclampsia has been reported in an adrenalectomized patient.[444] These two studies suggest that aldosterone does not play a role in the development of preeclampsia. The suppressed aldosterone secretion seen in preeclampsia may be secondary to sodium and fluid retention from another mechanism. It has been proposed that diminished progesterone and urinary pregnanediol in preeclampsia may result in less inhibition of aldosterone at the distal tubule, which results in sodium retention,[442, 445] but the decrease in aldosterone secretion is proportionately greater than the fall in progesterone secretion, and both may be diminished secondary to salt retention.[437] Esterogen secretion by the placenta also decreases in patients with preeclampsia.[446, 447, 448]

Studies of the renin-angiotensin system in subjects with preeclampsia have yielded conflicting results; renin activity is shown to be up in one study[421] and down in another.[419] Renin concentration was found to be decreased in three studies[419, 427, 449] and elevated in one study.[426] Renin substrate[419] and angiotensin II levels[422] were increased in a single study each. The fall in renin concentration observed in most studies to date might well be another reflection of the excessive sodium and fluid retention that characterizes preeclampsia-eclampsia.

An attempt has been made to link the renin-angiotensin system to the pathophysiology of preeclampsia. In an experiment producing uterine ischemia with polyethylene cuffs around the uterine arteries of dogs before they mated, hypertension, proteinuria, and hypernatremia developed with pregnancy and resolved after delivery.[450] Uterine vein renin rises under these circumstances, and evidence has been presented implicating the fetal kidneys as the source of renin production.[451, 452, 453, 454] Because plasma renin concentration declines in most studies of patients with eclampsia, the relationship of this experimental model to human toxemia is not clear.

Elevated secretion of chorionic gonadotropin has also been reported in patients with eclampsia.[455,456] Subsequent studies have shown that this elevation is commonly associated with fetal death and premature delivery, even in the absence of preeclampsia.[457,458,459,460,461] Elevated levels of chorionic gonadotropin also have been reported in 15% of normal pregnancies.[462]

In patients with severe preeclampsia, elevated levels of urinary antidiuretic factors have been reported that are not found in mild preeclampsia or normal pregnant subjects. This increase appears to be in proportion to the degree of edema.[463] Antidiuretic hormone does not appear to be a major factor in the development of preeclampsia, since this disorder develops in patients with diabetes insipidus.[464]

PROSTAGLANDINS, THE KALLIKREIN-KININ SYSTEM, AND PREGNANCY

A large body of data relates the products of arachidonic metabolism in various tissues to the regulation of vascular resistance, blood pressure, renal function, and the renin-angiotensin system.[465] During pregnancy, the uterus actively synthesizes large amounts of PGE_2, a vasodilator with natriuretic properties.[466] Elevated uterine blood flow during pregnancy depends upon continued synthesis of PGE_2.[466] Plasma and urine levels of PGE_2 metabolites rise during normal pregnancy[467] (Fig 6–6). Pharmacologic agents that inhibit the cyclooxygenase step of prostaglandin synthesis, such as the nonsteroidal anti-inflammatory agents, have potentially adverse effects on the fetal circulation, leading to the premature closure of the ductus arteriosus and to the development of pulmonary hypertension.[468]

The concentration of PGE_2 in the uterine vein of pregnant rabbits is increased to levels of 750-fold higher than those found in the renal vein of nonpregnant rabbits.[467] Both plasma and urinary concentration of PGE_2 increases during the third trimester of pregnancy,[467] probably due to an increase in renal as well as uterine synthesis.[469] Inhibition of cyclooxygenase with nonsteroidal anti-inflammatory agents reduce uterine vein PGE_2 levels and uterine blood flow concomitantly.[468]

Prostaglandin I_2 synthesis also appears to be elevated during the last trimester of pregnancy, as plasma and urine levels of a metabolite, 6-oxo-prostaglandin $F_{1\alpha}$ (6-oxo-$PGF_{1\alpha}$) become elevated, and higher levels of this breakdown product are found in the canine uterine vein[470] than in peripheral blood. Further, the myometrium of human subjects has been found to synthesize PGI_2,[471] as have the placenta and umbilical vessels of human subjects.[472, 473] Increased PGI_2 synthesis might explain the decrease in sensitivity to infused angiotensin which occurs during a normal pregnancy, since indomethacin can increase sensitivity to infusions of angiotensin when given during the final trimester of pregnancy[474] as well as at other times (Fig 6–7). Since preeclampsia is characterized by a loss of the normal decrease in angiotensin sensitivity during pregnancy, it can be postulated that impaired prostaglandin synthesis plays a role in the pathogenesis of preeclampsia[475, 476] (see Fig 6–8). Prostacyclin or PGI_2, a vasodilator, has been infused intravenously to treat 1 patient with severe hypertension during pregnancy with good results, although a transient fall in fetal heart rate was

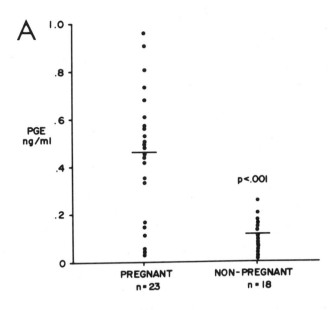

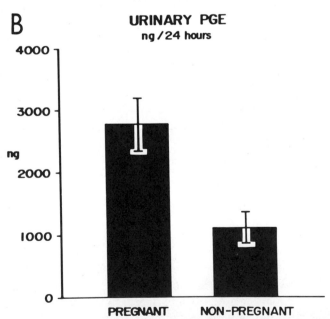

Fig 6–6.—**A,** peripheral venous prostaglandin E in third-trimester pregnant and in nonpregnant women. **B,** urinary prostaglandin secretion in pregnant and in nonpregnant women. (From Bay W.H., Ferris T.F.: Factors controlling plasma renin and aldosterone during pregnancy. *Hypertension* 1:410–415, 1979. Used by permission of the American Heart Association.)

noted.[477] However, in a recent study, Jouppila et al.[477a] noted that although intravenous infusion of PGI_2 lowered blood pressure in patients with pregnancy-induced hypertension, the reduction in pressure was accompanied by a slight reduction in uterine blood flow, suggesting that replacement of PGI_2 does not correct the impairment of uteroplacental blood flow that characteristically accompanies preeclampsia.

Several observations suggest that the kallikrein-kinin system is involved in the regulation of the uteroplacental circulation during pregnancy. A kallikrein-like enzyme in the human uterus and placenta has been described.[478] The plasma levels of kininogen rise during pregnancy[479, 480] and fall during labor.[481] Urinary kallikrein excretion rises during normal pregnancy[480] and falls to levels beneath those of a normal nonpregnant individual in patients who develop hypertension during pregnancy.[481] Infusion of bradykinin increases uterine blood flow.[482] Seino et al.[483] have demonstrated that inhibitors of kininase II

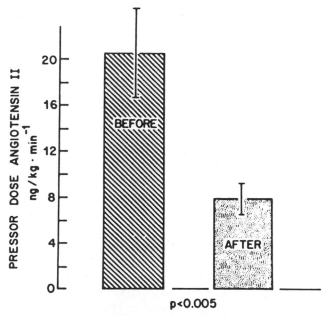

Fig 6–7.—The mean effective pressor dose of angiotensin II before and during indomethacin treatment of 11 normotensive women studied during late gestation. (From Everett R.B., et al.: Effect of prostaglandin synthetase inhibitors on pressor response to angiotensin II in human pregnancy. *J. Clin. Endocrinol. Metab.* 46:1007, 1978. Used by permission.)

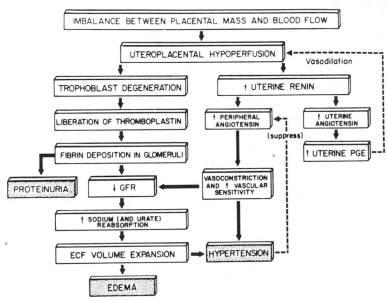

Fig 6–8.—A unified working hypothesis for the pathophysiology of pregnancy-induced hypertension. The *solid lines* lead to three primary manifestations: proteinuria, edema, and hypertension. The *dotted lines* indicate attempts to counteract the underlying defect of uteroplacental hypoperfusion. (From Kaplan N.M.: *Clinical Hypertension*, ed. 3. Baltimore, Williams & Wilkins Co., 1982, p. 367. Used by permission.)

increase uterine and placental blood flow in the rabbit without changes in systemic hemodynamics. Pretreatment with aprotinin or kinin antibodies blocked the increase in flow. Inhibition of converting enzyme also increased PGE_2 release, which was not seen after pretreatment with aprotinin, suggesting that the increase in flow might have been due to an effect of kinins on prostaglandin release, which has also been suggested by experiments showing that indomethacin reduces the increase in uterine blood flow induced by the administration of bradykinin.

Although present evidence suggests that the prostaglandins play an important role in normal pregnancies and in normal fetal development, much more must be known before disorders of prostaglandin and kinin metabolism can be implicated in the genesis of pregnancy-induced hypertension or before prostaglandins, kinins or compounds that influence their synthesis and catabolism can be used intelligently to treat these disorders.

HEMOSTASIS IN HYPERTENSIVE PREGNANCY

During normal pregnancy, a number of changes take place in four major areas concerned with the maintenance of hemostasis: the coagulation system, the blood platelet, the fibrinolytic system, and the vascular endothelium. Normal gestation is accompanied by an elevation of plasma levels of Factors VII, VIII, X, XIII, and fibrinogen,[484] changes which enhance coagulation. At the same time, levels of plasminogen activator fall, reducing the potency of the fibrinolytic system. In the late stages of pregnancy, Ylikorkala and Viinikka have found that blood platelets contain a higher content of thromboxane and have an enhanced tendency to aggregate.[485] During the same late phase of pregnancy, Lewis et al.[486] have found high plasma levels of 6-oxo-$PGF_{1\alpha}$, probably reflecting enhanced synthesis of antiaggregatory PGI_2 by vascular endothelium.

In preeclampsia, severe vasospasm is known to occur, which could disrupt the normal endothelial barrier to intravascular coagulation by exposing collagen, releasing tissue thromboplastin, and activating blood platelets as well as the intrinsic and extrinsic limbs of the coagulation cascade. Several observations indicate that mild intravascular coagulation takes place in preeclampsia. Factor VIII consumption is increased in preeclampsia and correlates with elevation of uric acid.[487] Weenink et al.[488] found decreased levels of antithrombin III in patients with pregnancy-induced and pregnancy-associated hypertension, but not in normal pregnancies, suggesting increased consumption in the hypertensive gravidas. Platelet counts decrease around mid pregnancy in women who later develop preeclampsia-eclampsia.[484] Maximum aggregation rates of platelets are decreased in toxemia,[489] which can be an indication of prior platelet aggregation. Several studies have found diminished synthesis of PGI_2 in the blood vessels of patients with preeclampsia-eclampsia and their infants.[490, 491, 492, 493] This observation could explain the vasospasm, platelet aggregation, and slow intravascular coagulation seen in patients with preeclampsia.

Urine and serum fibrin degradation products are increased in preeclampsia.[484] It has been observed that fibrin deposits are formed in the renal capillary loops and liver in cases of severe eclampsia. These studies suggest that intravascular coagulation plays a role in the pathogenesis of preeclampsia-eclampsia. Faith and Trump have demonstrated that the endothelial cells of the glomerular capillaries act as phagocytes and ingest fibrin.[494] Fibrin deposits have been observed within the glomerular capillary endothelial cells and along the basement membrane in patients with preclampsia. Using immunofluorescent methods, early investigators were unable to demonstrate deposits of immunoglobulins or complement within the glomerular endothelial cells, as are seen in lupus erythematosis and glomerulonephritis.[495] This initially suggested that immunologic injury does not play a role in the renal lesion. However, in a 1974 study of renal biopsy specimens from 11 patients with preeclampsia, Petrucco et al.[496] observed glomerular deposits of immunoglobulin and complement, providing evidence that the immune system is involved in preeclampsia. Renal lesions resembling those of preeclampsia have been produced in rabbits by the infusion of thromboplastin. This intervention presumably results in the formation of fibrin, which is then phagocytosed by the endothelial cells of the glomerular capillaries and by other cells of the reticuloendothelial system.[495] It is possible that uptake of fibrin by endothelial cells renders them more susceptible to damage.

Feeding oxidized cod-liver oil to pregnant rats causes intravascular coagulation with pathologic changes resembling those seen in human preeclampsia but without producing hypertension, proteinuria, or edema.[496] This process can be prevented by blockade of the reticuloendothelial system with tocopherol, which suggests that the accumulation of oxidants in tissues throughout the body results in cell membrane damage and secondary intravascular coagulation.

The generalized Schwartzman reaction can initiate disseminated intravascular coagulation and can be produced by the injection of endotoxin into rats who are in late pregnancy but not in mid pregnancy.[497] In one study, endotoxin caused deposits of fibrin in the glomerular capillaries and abortion in 56% of the experimental animals.[498] It is possible that placental injury from a number of causes could result in the release of thromboplastin, causing disseminated intravascular coagulation, glomerular fibrin deposition, and the syndrome of preeclampsia-eclampsia in human subjects.[499] Fortunately, clinically apparent disseminated intravascular coagulation is a relatively rare complication and is seen in no more than 3% of cases of severe preeclampsia-eclampsia.[500]

MAGNESIUM AND CALCIUM

For decades, magnesium sulfate has been an important part of the therapy for severe preeclampsia and eclampsia because of its capacity to reduce central nervous system irritability significantly and to lower blood pressure somewhat. Elevation of blood magnesium levels reduces arterial and venous tone and reduces drug-induced increases of tone.[501, 505] When the magnesium content of solutions bathing isolated arterial strips is lowered rapidly, a contractile response is elicited,[502] and the vessels become more reactive to angiotensin II, bradykinin, serotonin, and $PGF_{2\alpha}$. Abrupt lowering of blood magnesium levels in pregnancy is followed by an increase in blood pressure accompanied by a rise in peripheral vascular resistance in animals and in humans.[503] Rats receiving a magnesium-deficient diet for 12 weeks developed elevated blood pressure which was accompanied by attenuation of the microcirculation.[504] Blood vessels have been found to contain magnesium sites which regulate the passage of calcium in and out of the cell.[505] When serum magnesium levels fell, intracellular calcium concentration rises, which, in contractile cells, increases vascular tone.

Hypomagnesemia has been found in patients with preeclampsia.[503, 506] Epidemiologic surveys have uncovered evidence that pregnant women have been ingesting less dietary magnesium over the past several decades.[503] The serum levels of magnesium have been found to decline during the final 2 months of gestation, even in nonhypertensive pregnancies.[507, 508] The placentas of patients with preeclampsia and eclampsia have been found to have decreased levels of magnesium and increased calcium concentration,[503, 509] which could lead to increased vascular resistance within the placenta, which could explain the uteroplacental ischemia that has been observed in preeclampsia.[336, 337, 338]

Population studies have found an inverse relationship between the calcium content of drinking water and mean blood pressure.[510, 511] Subsequent studies, which rely on dietary histories, have found that hypertensive subjects ingest less calcium, among other nutrients, than normotensive subjects,[512] while other studies have found the opposite. A Belgian study[513] of more than 9,000 military personnel found blood pressure to be directly related to serum calcium levels. Calcium restriction has been found to elevate blood pressure in the rat,[514, 515, 516] while calcium supplements have been found to lower blood pressure in the rat[517, 518] and in some human subjects.[519]

In pregnant rats, calcium restriction has caused an elevation of blood pressure that reverses when calcium intake is restored.[518] Since growth of the fetal skeleton increases calcium requirements during pregnancy,[520] one can postulate that an adequate calcium intake might be important in preventing the development of hypertension during pregnancy.

Epidemiologic studies have uncovered data suggesting that calcium deficiency is associated with eclampsia. The low incidence of eclampsia in Guatemala, despite circumstances which might be predicted to lead to a high frequency, led to a study of the incidence of eclampsia in three countries with varying levels of calcium intake.[521] In Guatemala and in the United States, where the average intake of calcium is high, a relatively low incidence of eclampsia was found. In contrast, the incidence of eclampsia was high, and dietary calcium intake low, in Colombia, even when adjusted for age, parity, and amount of prenatal care, factors known to be associated with preeclampsia-eclampsia.

While the interpretation of these data remain a matter of controversy, since free cytosolic calcium usually increases the tension of vascular tissue[522] and might be expected to increase blood pressure, as is often the case in patients with hyperparathyroidism[523] or acute elevation of serum calcium,[524] sufficient evidence has been presented that dietary calcium intake is in some way involved in the control of blood pressure to warrant further serious study of the problem.

HELMINTHS AND PREECLAMPSIA

In 1983 Lueck et al.[525] reported their observations of a worm-like structure in the blood of patients with preeclampsia or gestational trophoblastic disease, which they concluded was helminthic in nature and a possible cause of preeclampsia. The putative organism was tentatively designated *Hydatoxi luaba*. Human placenta containing these structures were concentrated and used to innoculate pregnant beagles, resulting in a toxemia-like syndrome characterized by hypertension with retinopathy, proteinuria, disseminated intravascular coagulation, hepatic dysfunction, intrauterine growth retardation, and fetal death. Autopsy showed glomeruloendotheliosis and hepatic periportal hemorrhage, lesions typically found in patients with preeclampsia.[526] Increased sensitivity to angiotensin II was also noted. Inoculation with placental concentrates that did not contain the helminth-like structures did not cause the toxemia-like syndrome.

Subsequently, Gau et al.[527] carried out electron microscopic examination of the organism, which they obtained by applying Lueck's staining technique to normal placenta and to the blood of normal men and concluded that the structures were not helminthic in nature. Further,

Richards, Grimes, and Wilson[528] at the Helminthic Diseases Branch of the Center for Disease Control have identified these vermiform struc-tures in toluidine blue O-stained smears of venous or cord blood from both patients with and without preeclampsia and from healthy beagle dogs. They found that the structures could not be concentrated by passing the blood through filter with a pore size of 12μ, even though the structures had a diameter of 30 to 670μ. In addition, the structures did not stain with Giemsa, which ordinarily demonstrates metazoan parasites, and the structures were pleomorphic, which is not a char-acteristic of helminths. Therefore, Richards and his colleagues con-cluded that the worm-like structures were probably an artifact of staining.

THE IMMUNE RESPONSE AND PREECLAMPSIA

Several observations have led to the hypothesis that preeclampsia has an immunologic basis.[529] This disorder tends to occur during a first pregnancy, which suggests the possibility that there is insufficient for-mation of blocking antibodies as antigenic sites develop on the pla-centa, thereby provoking an immune response against a placenta per-ceived as immunologically incompatible with maternal tissues. An anamnestic response would explain the formation of adequate quanti-ties of blocking antibodies during subsequent pregnancies. In 1978 Beer[529] analyzed the various clinical and experimental observations as-sociated with preeclampsia-eclampsia and pointed out that an immu-nologic hypothesis could explain not only the tendency of this disorder to occur in primiparas and the subsequent protection afforded by a first pregnancy, but also the decreased incidence in cosanguineous mar-riages, the increased incidence in immunosuppressed patients, the in-creased incidence in pregnancies with a large placenta, with cure fol-lowing the delivery of the placenta, the pathologic changes that occur in the placenta and kidneys, and the association with disseminated in-travascular coagulation. However, Beer concluded that the unique as-sociation with human patients, the hypertension, edema, and convul-sions, and the familial link with nutritional deficiencies are difficult or impossible to explain on an immune basis.

Subsequent work has extended these considerations. It is now documented that maternal recognition of fetal antigen actually takes place[530] and that the formation of maternal antibodies directed against fetal antigens occur during most pregnancies. Binding of maternal antibodies to fetal antigens takes place at the placental level and probably results in activation of the complement system, although incontestable proof of the latter is still lacking, as studies have demonstrated an increase in levels of Clq, C4, C3, and CH5 in normal pregnancy and an absence of complement activators.[530] However, in recent immunologic studies of human placenta from normal and preeclamptic pregnancies, Sinha, Wells, and Faulk[531] found increased deposition of Clq, C3d, and C9 in preeclampsia. Further, the degree of increase correlated with the severity of chorionic villus immunopathology when cases of mild and severe preeclampsia were compared, providing additional evidence that an immune process was involved in the pathophysiology of preeclampsia. Anderson[532] points out that the interposed tissues of the placenta serve as important filters with temporal morphological features whose relevance remains to be established. He further stated that new techniques were needed to determine the importance of transplacental antigen traffic. One such step has recently been reported by O'-Sullivan et al.,[533] who developed an immunoradiometric technique for the detection of human trophoblast-specific membrane antigen in maternal blood during pregnancy and demonstrated such antigens in the blood of pregnant women but not in that of men or nonpregnant women. When they applied their method to the study of preeclampsia, they found no differences, suggesting that differential trophoblast antigen deposition does not play a role in the etiology of preeclampsia. Antigens were also measured in samples of retroplacental cord blood from normal and preeclamptic pregnancies; results ranged from negative to barely detectable, suggesting that the deposition of trophoblast membrane antigen was limited to the maternal side of the placenta. Masson et al.[534] found immune complexes in the serum of 54 normal pregnant women and proposed that the complexes acted to block placental rejection. Stirrat et al.[535] found higher levels of immune complex in 16 patient with preeclampsia compared to 16 control subjects, and D'Amelio et al.[536] found elevated levels in only 2 of 10 preeclamptic subjects. However, the levels fell with delivery, suggesting that they were involved in the disease process.

Persitz et al.[537] have examined the antigens of the major histocompatibility complex in normal and severely preeclamptic pregnancies and found no differences. These data suggest that histocompatibility is not involved in the susceptibility to severe preeclampsia.

Several recent studies have investigated the possibility that circulating immune complexes play a role in the pathogenesis of preeclampsia. Medcalf et al.[538] found levels of circulating immune complex greater than 20 g/ml heat-aggregated IgG in 14 of 20 patients with preeclampsia and in 6 of 19 normal subjects. As concentrations in this range have been shown to activate the release reaction of human platelets in vitro, it is possible that these complexes are involved in the development of intravascular coagulation and vasospasm in preeclampsia.[539] V'ázquez-Escobosa et al.[540] found evidence of circulating immune complexes in 20 patients with preeclampsia-eclampsia, using the method of phagocytosis and immunofluorescence. These were composed of IgG and C3 and were not found in normal pregnancy, or pregnancy accompanying essential or renal hypertension. Using the Raji cell test, Kuramoto et al.[541] demonstrated circulating immune complexes in patients with preeclampsia which did not correlate with clinical symptoms at 29 to 31 weeks but became strongly correlated at 29 to 31 weeks and just before delivery. Schena et al.[542] demonstrated that circulating immune complexes are low in the first trimester of normal pregnancy and show further decrease as the pregnancy progresses. In contrast, circulating immune complexes are higher in women who develop preeclampsia, increase with exacerbation of symptoms, and fall after delivery. During the same study, measurements of the various components of the complement system failed to reveal a difference between normal and preeclamptic pregnancies.

Not all studies have yielded evidence of increased circulating immune complexes during preeclampsia. Rote and Caudle[543] used a Raji cell enzyme-linked immunoabsorbent assay and polyethylene glycol precipitation methods to study 86 subjects and did not observe circulating immune complexes in normal or preeclamptic pregnant subjects. Similar negative results have been reported by Knox et al.[544] and Pudifin et al.[545]

The possibility that cell-mediated immunity is involved in the pathogenesis of preeclampsia has been explored in a number of recent studies. A variety of abnormalities have been described. Alanen and Lassila[546] examined the in vitro response of maternal lymphocytes to phytohemagglutinin, concanavalin, and purified protein derivative of tuberculin. Although responses were lower in pregnant than in nonpregnant subjects, there were no significant differences between normal gravidas and those with preeclampsia. However, the number of active E rosette-forming cells was higher in the blood of preeclamptic patients. In separate studies, they also found evidence of reduced killer cell activity in the lymphocytes of 15 patients with preeclampsia, as compared to normal pregnant and nonpregnant women.[547]

Moore et al.[548] studied lymphocyte subsets in normal and preeclamptic pregnancies using monoclonal antibodies to OKT3, OKT4, and OKT8 cells. While no differences between normal pregnant and nonpregnant subjects were found, 10 preeclamptic patients were found to have a significant increase in OKT4-positive helper cells. However, Gusdon et al.[549] performed similar studies in 11 normal and 10 preeclamptic subjects, measuring OKM1, OKT3, OKT4, OKT8, OKT11, and OKla and found instead that the only significant change was a significant decrease in OKM1 populations in the third trimester of normal pregnancy, which was not observed in preeclamptic subjects.

Taufield et al.[550] examined cellular responsiveness and hormonal suppressor activity in normal and preeclamptic pregnancies. Using mixed lymphocyte culture reactions, they found that maternal lymphocytes were hyporesponsive to fetal cells but not to unrelated control cells. Serum from normal pregnant subjects suppressed lymphocytes when maternal cells were responder cells and maternal or fetal cells were stimulator cells. In contrast, neither lymphocytes nor serum from preeclamptic patients demonstrated cellular hyperresponsiveness or humeral suppressor activity. The authors speculate that suppression of maternal-fetal immunity appears to characterize normal pregnancies, and may make them possible, while impairment of this adaptive immunity could be a cause of preeclampsia. In related studies, Sargent et al.[551] have studied maternal-paternal mixed lymphocyte reactivity in normal and preeclamptic pregnancies and found differences which might reflect an abnormal immune response.

Sridama et al.[552] used monoclonal anti-T-cell antibodies to study peripheral blood mononuclear cells from patients with preeclampsia and found that the percentage of total T cells was significantly reduced in such patients, compared to those with normal pregnancies.

In a unique study, Pietarinen et al.[553] have used indirect immunofluorescence to detect smooth muscle antibodies in the sera of patients with hypertensive disorders of pregnancy and have found an increased incidence in patients with preeclampsia. However, smooth muscle antibodies were also found in pregnant patients with edema or intrahepatic cholestasis, indicating the abnormality is not specific and suggesting that it is a result, rather than a cause, of the disorder.

Thus, clues abound that abnormalities of the immune system are present in preeclampsia. However, many of the reports are conflicting and many have not been confirmed. While the weight of evidence currently suggests that circulating immune complexes are found in the blood of patients with preeclampsia, variation in experimental technique and several conflicting reports prevent one from concluding with certainty that the complexes are involved in the pathogenesis of this disorder. Resolution of the question awaits the development of better techniques and additional studies.

CHAPTER 7

CONSEQUENCES OF ELEVATED BLOOD PRESSURE

IN ORDER TO evolve a rationale for treating patients with blood pressure elevation, one must examine the effects of hypertension on the cardio-vascular system that lead to the development of vascular disease (Fig 7–1). Since the development in 1896 of methods for clinical measure-ment of blood pressure,[554] extensive data have been collected. During the next 60 years, patients were followed without effective antihyper-tensive therapy. It was soon clear that severely elevated blood pressure was associated with a grave prognosis. Patients with diastolic blood pressure of 130 mm Hg and above had a short time to survive when the elevated pressure was associated with evidence of significant dam-age of target organs: papilledema, retinal hemorrhages and exudates, congestive heart failure, or diminished renal function. The most fre-quent symptoms in such patients were visual impairment, headache, gross hematuria, dyspnea, edema, nausea, vomiting, epigastric pain, and malaise.[555] In one series of 105 cases, it was noted that most pa-tients died within 4 months, and that few patients survived longer than 16 months.[556] In these patients, the malignant phase of elevated blood pressure was associated most often with either essential or renal parenchymal hypertension. In a series of 124 cases studied postmor-tem, chronic pyelonephritis was found in 21%, and chronic glomeru-lonephritis in 15%.[557]

With the development of effective treatment, it became apparent that prognosis was improved by the use of antihypertensive agents. The results of several studies suggested that antihypertensive therapy

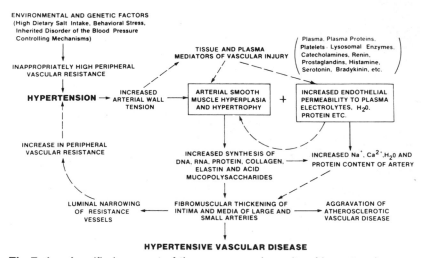

ENVIRONMENTAL AND GENETIC FACTORS
(High Dietary Salt Intake, Behavioral Stress,
Inherited Disorder of the Blood Pressure
Controlling Mechanisms)

TISSUE AND PLASMA
MEDIATORS OF VASCULAR INJURY

Plasma, Plasma Proteins,
Platelets · Lysosomal Enzymes,
Catecholamines, Renin,
Prostaglandins, Histamine,
Serotonin, Bradykinin, etc.

INAPPROPRIATELY HIGH PERIPHERAL
VASCULAR RESISTANCE

HYPERTENSION → INCREASED ARTERIAL WALL TENSION → ARTERIAL SMOOTH MUSCLE HYPERPLASIA AND HYPERTROPHY + INCREASED ENDOTHELIAL PERMEABILITY TO PLASMA ELECTROLYTES, H_2O, PROTEIN ETC.

INCREASE IN PERIPHERAL
VASCULAR RESISTANCE

INCREASED SYNTHESIS OF
DNA, RNA, PROTEIN, COLLAGEN,
ELASTIN AND ACID
MUCOPOLYSACCHARIDES

INCREASED Na^+, Ca^{2+}, H_2O AND
PROTEIN CONTENT OF ARTERY

LUMINAL NARROWING
OF RESISTANCE
VESSELS

FIBROMUSCULAR THICKENING OF
INTIMA AND MEDIA OF LARGE AND
SMALL ARTERIES

AGGRAVATION OF
ATHEROSCLEROTIC
VASCULAR DISEASE

HYPERTENSIVE VASCULAR DISEASE

Fig 7–1.—A unified concept of the causes and results of hypertensive vascular disease. (From Hollander W.: Role of hypertension in atherosclerosis and cardiovascular disease. *Am. J. Cardiol.* 38:786, 1976. Used by permission.)

lengthened the half-time of survival of patients with malignant hypertension from approximately 6 months to about 2½ years. Patients with prior renal damage did not show as great an improvement in survival with treatment as did patients with well-preserved renal function, because of progression of underlying renal disease.[558] Improved prognosis was limited by renal damage or underlying renal parenchymal disease. Patients with impaired renal function, i.e., endogenous creatinine clearance of less than 45 ml/min, did not do as well with treatment. Only 4 out of 15 patients with less than this clearance were alive 1 year after the initiation of therapy, whereas 8 of 11 patients with more than this clearance were alive 1 year after beginning therapy.[559] The prognosis for these patients has been improved by the increasing availability of hemodialysis, which allows support of renal function while renal blood flow falls transiently as arterial pressure is lowered.[560]

Hodge and Smirk noted that treated hypertensive patients ultimately died from complications that differed from those responsible for the deaths of untreated patients.[561] Prior to the era of antihypertensive therapy, 32% of hypertensive patients died with cerebral vascular accidents, 22% from congestive heart failure, 21% from coronary artery disease, 1.4% from uremia, and 24% from other causes. After the development of antihypertensive therapy, 42% of patients died from coronary disease, 23% from cerebral vascular accidents, 9.5% from uremia, 6% from congestive heart failure, and 20% from other causes.

These data suggest that partial control of severe hypertension improved prognosis, but those patients who had residual blood pressure elevation continued to develop target-organ damage. The findings indicated additional study of the adverse effects of less severe levels of blood pressure elevation. In 1959, the Build and Blood Pressure Study of the United States Society of Actuaries pointed out that blood pressure and longevity were inversely related, starting at levels of around 90/60 mm Hg.[562] These observations were confirmed by the study of 1979.[563]

In 1954, the residents of Framingham, Massachusetts, were invited to participate in a long-term study of cardiovascular morbidity and mortality.[564] This investigation was observational, and no therapeutic interventions were initiated. The participants underwent physical and laboratory examination followed by reevaluation at 2-year intervals. Of the 5,127 men and women between 30 and 60 years of age who entered the study, 18% of the men and 16% of the women had systolic blood pressures greater than 160 or diastolic pressures greater than 95 mm Hg. Forty-one percent of the men had blood pressure elevations above 140 systolic and 90 mm Hg diastolic while 48% of the women were in this range. For patients with moderate elevation of blood pressure, the risk of developing congestive heart failure was found to be six times greater than in subjects with a blood pressure lower than 140/90. The risk of developing a stroke was three to five times as great and the risk of having a fatal heart attack was two to three times as great. The higher the blood pressure, the shorter was the life expectancy. The risk of developing cardiovascular disease was incremental, increasing with the level of blood pressure. These observations applied to women as well as to men, were independent of age at the time of initial examination, and applied even when other risk factors, such as abnormal lipids, obesity, diabetes, and ECG abnormalities were considered. Deaths in hypertensive patients were due to severe cardiovascular disorders: atherothrombotic brain infarction, coronary heart disease, congestive heart failure, hemorrhagic and nonhemorrhagic stroke. Cerebral vascular accidents were a greater cause of death and disability among hypertensive women than among hypertensive men.[565] In malignant hypertension, death usually occurs from uremia and cerebral hemorrhage, with male and female patients sharing the risk equally. With moderate hypertension, the major risks are morbidity and mortality from coronary heart disease and hemorrhagic and thrombotic cerebrovascular accidents.

Data collected by the National Health Examination Survey of the Public Health Service on a random sample of the adult United States population between the ages of 18 and 79 years showed that 16% of white adults and 30% of black adults had diastolic blood pressures higher than 90 mm Hg.[566] When a diastolic pressure of 95 mm Hg is used as a cutoff point, 9% of white adults and 22% of black adults are found to be above this level. This survey revealed that the prevalence of hypertension was roughly two times as high in blacks as in whites. When hypertension was found in blacks, blood pressure levels tended to be higher than in whites. As a consequence, hypertensive heart disease was present from three to nine times more frequently in various subgroups of the black population than in comparable white subgroups.[567]

There is evidence to indicate that it is elevation of blood pressure itself that causes vascular complications. In experimental animals, induced vasoconstriction is followed by sclerotic changes within the arterioles and necrosis of surrounding tissues.[568] In man, three observations indicate that atherosclerotic changes are related to the level of blood pressure. In patients with coarctation of the aorta, atherosclerotic lesions are found in the high-pressure area of the aorta but not in the low-pressure area beyond the coarctation.[569] Patients with congenital heart disease and with long-standing pulmonary hypertension develop atherosclerotic lesions in the pulmonary arterial tree.[570] In patients with renal artery stenosis and associated hypertension, nephrosclerotic changes develop in the "healthy kidney," whereas the vascular tree distal to the stenosis in the ischemic kidney is usually protected from the development of nephrosclerosis.[571] The complications of hypertension are directly related to the level of the high blood pressure, but the risk imposed by a given level of arterial pressure is increased by the concomitant presence of additional risk factors: smoking, hypercholesterolemia, diabetes mellitus, and a family history of cardiovascular disease.

RATIONALE FOR TREATMENT

The goal in treating a patient with hypertension is to prevent the premature development of cardiovascular disease. The complications related to high blood pressure per se are: further progression of hypertension, renal failure, hemorrhagic stroke, congestive heart failure, and dissecting aneurysm. Other complications are related to the accelerated atherosclerosis associated with hypertension: acute myocardial infarction, atherothrombotic cerebral infarction, and intermittent claudication. Even patients with minimal blood pressure elevation are subject to the development of these atheromatous complications.

Almost three decades ago, it was found that antihypertensive medications prevented the development of necrotic and sclerotic changes in the arterioles of animals with experimental hypertension.[572] In clinical use, it became apparent that patients with accelerated or malignant hypertension could benefit from therapy;[573, 574] however, it was not known whether patients with diastolic blood pressures between 90 and 129 mm Hg had anything to gain from the expense and inconvenience of chronic antihypertensive therapy or whether the risks of therapy outweighed the benefits of lowering blood pressure. In 1964, Hamilton, Thompson, and Wisniewski[575] reported the results of an 8-year prospective study which found that only 4% of an effectively treated group of hypertensive patients developed the complications of hypertension. In 1966, Wolff and Lindeman[576] reported a controlled 2-year study of 87 patients which also showed only 33% as many cardiovascular complications in a treated group as in a group receiving placebo.

The next major study of this problem was the Veterans Administration Cooperative Study of Antihypertensive Agents.[577, 578] In this project, male veterans were hospitalized for an evaluation which excluded those with diastolic blood pressure above 129 mm Hg, those with secondary hypertension, and those whose blood pressure dropped beneath 90 mm Hg without therapy. Patients who already had evidence of cardiovascular complications were included in the trial. After a placebo lead-in period, the patients were randomized blindly into two groups. One group received placebo and the other group received hydrochlorothiazide, with reserpine and then hydralazine added stepwise as needed.

It soon became apparent that the subgroup of patients with the highest blood pressures were developing complications rapidly. As a result, the 143 patients who entered the study with diastolic blood pressures between 115 and 129 mm Hg were analyzed after a period of about 20 months. Analysis of events in the untreated group showed that 7 patients had developed grade three to four retinopathy; 3, accelerated hypertension; 3, renal failure; 3, dissecting aneurysm; 2, retinopathy with congestive heart failure; 2, strokes; 1, sudden death; 2, myocardial infarction; 2, congestive heart failure; and 2, minor strokes. In contrast, 1 patient in the treated group developed a drug reaction and 1 patient suffered a minor stroke. The difference between the two groups was highly significant, and it was proved that antihypertensive therapy benefited male patients with a diastolic blood pressure between 115 and 129 mm Hg.

This left a subgroup of 380 patients who had entered the study with average, resting diastolic pressures between 90 and 114 mm Hg during the initial hospitalization. These patients were followed for as long as 5 years, with an average follow-up of 3.3 years. There were 35 terminating morbid events in the control group as opposed to 9 in the treated group, 21 nonterminating cardiovascular events in the control group as opposed to 13 in the treated group, and 20 instances of accelerated hypertension in the control group as opposed to none in the treated group. The fatalities consisted of 7 strokes in the control group and none in the treated group, 3 myocardial infarctions in the control group and 2 in the treated group, 8 instances of sudden death in the control group as opposed to 4 in the treated group, and 1 instance of ruptured arteriosclerotic aneurysm in the treated group. There were 12 nonfatal strokes in the control group and only 1 in the treated group, 11 cases of coronary heart disease in the control group and 6 in the treated group, 5 cases of congestive failure in the control group and none in the treated group, 4 cases of accelerated hypertension in the control group as opposed to 9 in the treated group, and 1 instance of renal damage in the control group and none in the treated group.

In analyzing the data from the subgroup of patients with diastolic blood pressure between 90 and 114 mm Hg, it was found that the risk of developing a morbid cardiovascular event during a 5-year period was reduced from 55% in the group receiving a placebo to only 18% in the group getting active treatment.[579] The difference between the treated and untreated group was statistically significant for patients with initial diastolic blood pressures of 105 mm Hg or more. For those patients who entered the trial with lower pressures, the risk of developing a cardiovascular event was not as great, and the benefit from antihypertensive therapy was not as marked, although the patients in this subgroup also appeared to benefit from treatment. In no instance did it appear that antihypertensive therapy increased morbidity or mortality, and indeed this study suggests that long-term antihypertensive therapy is relatively benign.

The Veterans Administration (VA) study established that treatment of male patients with a diastolic blood pressure above 105 mm Hg conveys significant benefit to the patient. Women were not studied. Thus, there was no proof that they would benefit equally from therapy. Physicians remained cautious about applying the results of this trial for several reasons. The starting blood pressures were defined as the average of the resting diastolic pressures from the fourth through the sixth day of hospitalization. Patients with significant levels of diastolic hypertension, when placed in the hospital, often become normotensive or nearly so by the fourth day. Thus, those patients participating in the VA study probably had more sustained hypertension. Secondly, although patients with mild blood pressure elevation are at risk of developing cardiovascular damage, they have less risk than patients with higher levels of blood pressure. The VA study showed that patients with levels of diastolic blood pressure between 90 and 104 mm Hg benefited less from antihypertensive therapy than their counterparts with higher blood pressures. Thus, when treating patients with mild elevations of blood pressure, it was advisable to weigh the limited benefit of therapy against the greater inconvenience, greater expense, and greater risk of side effects from antihypertensive therapy. The risk-benefit ratio in this group is not as favorable as it is in those individuals who have a persistent diastolic blood pressure above 105 mm Hg.

In the mid 1970s, considering the data from the Build and Blood Pressure Study, from Framingham, from the VA studies and from other sources, many authorities conservatively recommended that patients with sustained diastolic blood pressures ranging from 90 mm Hg to 104 mm Hg receive treatment based on individual consideration. A very important factor in reaching a decision to prescribe antihypertensive medications for such patients was the presence or absence of additional cardiovascular risk factors. As these factors appear to be additive, a patient with a slight risk imposed by a minor elevation of blood pressure has a much greater chance of developing cardiovascular disease if he or she also smokes cigarettes, has diabetes mellitus, elevated serum cholesterol, or has a family history of premature cardiovascular disease. In such a case, an attempt should be made to reduce as many risk factors as possible, including the elevated blood pressure.

The results of the Veterans Administration study have been extended in an important way by the recent findings of the Hypertension Detection and Follow-up Program (HDFP), a 5-year, fourteen-center study involving 10,900 patients, which provided the first convincing evidence that mortality in patients with a diastolic blood pressure of 90 to 104 mm Hg was reduced by effective antihypertensive therapy.[580]

The participants in HDFP ranged in age from 30 to 69 years of age and included both men and women. Over 70% of the cohort had diastolic blood pressures between 90 and 104 mm Hg. The patients were stratified on the basis of age, sex, race, organ involvement, and prior treatment history and were randomized into one of two groups. One group received treatment from their usual source of medical care, the other received intensive antihypertensive therapy at special centers where free medications were given, waiting time was short, extensive patient education measures were used, and lost patients were retrieved. Stepped-care therapy was used, consisting of thiazide diuretic, with the addition of reserpine, methyldopa, or, less frequently, propranolol, if needed. Hydralazine, then guanethidine were added in sequence if goal blood pressure had not been reached. The therapeutic goal of the centers was to lower diastolic blood pressure to levels beneath 90 mm Hg or by 10 mm Hg, whichever figure was lowest. By the end of 5 years, the goal had been achieved in 64.9% of the center-care patients and in 43.6% of the referred-care group. Thus, both groups received antihypertensive treatment. The difference lay in the effectiveness. Although the average starting diastolic blood pressure was about 101 mm Hg in both groups, after 5 years, blood pressure had fallen to 84.1 mm Hg in the center-care group, while falling to 89.1 mm Hg in the referred-care patients. Mortality from all causes was 17% lower in the center-care group; 20% lower in patients whose pretreatment diastolic pressure was 90–104 mm Hg. The difference was highly significant ($P < .01$). Similarly, effective treatment reduced deaths from cerebrovascular disease by 45% and deaths from acute myocardial infarction by 46%. Overall, there was a 15% reduction in the death rate from ischemic heart disease in the center-care group.

Similarly, an Australian trial of therapy in 3,427 patients with mild hypertension has demonstrated the beneficial effect of treatment of individuals whose pretreatment diastolic blood pressure ranged between 95 and 109 mm Hg.[581] In this trial, mortality from cardiovascular disease was reduced by two thirds over a 4-year period. This trial included a blinded control group treated with placebo, which makes its conclusions particularly convincing. The existence of the placebo group made possible the interesting observation that fully 45% of placebo-treated patients experienced a fall in diastolic pressure to levels beneath 95 mm Hg over a 3-year period.

Thus, there is now strong evidence to support the benefit of lowering blood pressure in asymptomatic individuals with diastolic blood pressure between 90–95 and 104 mm Hg, even if they are free of end-organ damage and even if they are relatively old (some of the participants in HDFP were aged 74 years at its conclusion). For those individuals with deceptively "mild" hypertension, treatment might appropriately begin with weight reduction, salt restriction, and regular exercise, with pharmacologic agents added when these measures are unsuccessful.

CHAPTER 8

CONSEQUENCES OF ELEVATED BLOOD PRESSURE DURING PREGNANCY

THE RESULTS OF the Collaborative Perinatal Project,[582] which examined fetal mortality in relationship to maximum diastolic pressure in 38,636 pregnancies, found that fetal mortality increased significantly when maternal diastolic pressure climbed above 95 mm Hg or fell beneath 64 mm Hg (Fig 8–1). When proteinuria was present, mortality was significantly higher among the fetuses of pregnant patients with diastolic pressures greater than 85 mm Hg. Similarly, in a prospective study of 14,833 women, Page and Christianson[583] have examined the course of pregnancy relative to blood pressure. Measurements of blood pressure were recorded during the fifth and sixth months of gestation. With each 5 mm Hg of rise in mean arterial pressure, there was a stepwise increase in perinatal mortality, which was higher in black subjects than in whites for a given level of pressure. A mean arterial pressure of 90 mm Hg or more during the middle trimester of pregnancy was associated with a significant increase in the rate of stillbirth, the incidence of preeclampsia, and the development of intrauterine fetal growth retardation. The unfavorable outcome was attributed to impairment of the uteroplacental circulation, which is known to be associated with hypertension.[584] They concluded that women with a mean blood pressure of 90 mm Hg or more during the fifth and sixth month of pregnancy constitute a high-risk group.[583]

A somewhat different experience was reported by Sibai, Abdella,

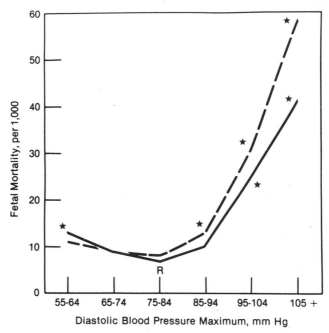

Fig 8–1.—Fetal mortality in relation to the maximal diastolic blood pressure recorded during 38,636 pregnancies by the Collaborative Perinatal Project. The *solid line* represents the total series; the *broken line* represents the patients with concomitant proteinuria of any degree. *Asterisks* designate mortality significantly higher than in patients with normal maximal diastolic values *(R)*. (From Friedman E.A., Neff R.K.: Hypertension-hypotension in pregnancy. Correlation with fetal outcome. *J.A.M.A.* 239:2249, 1978. Used by permission; copyright 1978, American Medical Association.)

and Anderson,[585] who followed the pregnancies of 211 patients whose diastolic blood pressure varied between 90 and 110 mm Hg prepartum. At the first prenatal visit, chronic antihypertensive therapy was discontinued. Thirteen percent of the patients eventually required reinstitution of therapy. There were 6 perinatal fetal deaths, 5 of which occurred among the 21 patients who developed superimposed preeclampsia. Thirty-two percent of the infants delivered by the preeclamptic mothers had retarded growth. In contrast, only 5.3% of the infants delivered by the others were retarded in growth and only 1 died. In those previously mildly hypertensive patients who did not develop preeclampsia, perinatal mortality approached that of the general obstetrical population. Other writers as well have concluded the maternal risk of mild chronic hypertension is relatively small, unless preeclampsia also develops, and may be no greater than that of nonhypertensive gravidas.[586, 587]

Table 8–1 compares the few published studies of perinatal mortality in hypertensive gravidas who received early antihypertensive therapy with other series in which hypertension was not treated until maternal diastolic blood pressure exceeded 110 mm Hg. However, none of the trials used a randomized, double-blinded study protocol, most involved very few patients, and the reported perinatal mortality rates varied widely, regardless of treatment rendered. Therefore, scientifically valid conclusions cannot be derived from this data.

Unfortunately, a trial comparable to the Hypertension Detection and Follow-up Program has not been carried out to determine with certainty which pregnant patients should be treated.

TABLE 8–1.—PERINATAL OUTCOME IN TREATED WOMEN WITH
CHRONIC HYPERTENSION*

AUTHOR(S)	ANTIHYPERTENSIVE REGIMEN	NUMBER	DEATHS	DEATHS PER 1000
Landesman et al. (1957)	Reserpine	80	8	100
Harley (1966)	Hydralazine + reserpine	214	40	187
Kincaid-Smith et al. (1966)	Methyldopa	32	3	94
Leather et al. (1968)	Methyldopa + thiazide	23	0	0
Redman et al. (1976)	Methyldopa or hydralazine	101	1	10
Total		**450**	**52**	**116**

PERINATAL MORTALITY IN WOMEN WITH CHRONIC HYPERTENSION WHO WERE
NOT TREATED UNTIL DIASTOLIC PRESSURE EXCEEDED 110 MM HG

AUTHOR	NUMBER	DEATHS	DEATHS PER 1000
Harley (1966)	349	39	110
Leather et al. (1968)	24	2	83
Redman et al. (1976)	107	2	19
Chesley (1978)	593	19	32 (23.8)†
Curet (1979)	72	3	41 (14)
Whalley‡	533	20	38 (34)
Total	**1678**	**85**	**50.7**

*Modified from Gant N.F. Jr., Worley R.J.: *Hypertension in Pregnancy, Concepts and Management.* New York, Appleton-Century-Crofts, 1980.
†Corrected perinatal mortality rate.
‡Unpublished.

Chronic hypertension can be complicated by superimposed pre-eclampsia in 25% to 30% of cases. The diagnosis of preeclampsia is made when hypertension appears after the 20th week of pregnancy, accompanied by edema and proteinuria of more than 300 mg/day. The detection of superimposed preeclampsia can be difficult, since pressure is already elevated, edema can be found in 80% of normal pregnancies,[588] and proteinuria may be mild. The distinction is important, however, as the superimposition of preeclampsia is often associated with a rapidly deteriorating clinical course.[586] The diagnosis should be suspected when blood pressure rises more than 30/15 mm Hg above the individual's usual levels, or when serum uric acid levels rise. It is not clear why preeclampsia develops during pregnancies that are complicated by essential hypertension but, as discussed previously, it may be due to the fact that uteroplacental perfusion is reduced in chronically hypertensive patients who become pregnant, and an inadequate placental blood flow from any cause has been proposed to be an etiologic factor in preeclampsia.

PROGNOSIS OF PREGNANCY-INDUCED HYPERTENSION

A number of studies have followed patients after hypertensive pregnancies in an attempt to determine the eventual clinical course. The results of such studies are sometimes difficult to interpret because of a lack of convincing documentation that the patient actually had preeclampsia-eclampsia, or pregnancy-induced hypertension, rather than essential hypertension which became manifest during pregnancy, or hypertension secondary to renal parenchymal disease, such as chronic glomerulonephritis or pyelonephritis, as was frequently found in the renal biopsies of clinically preeclamptic patients.[390] Further, many earlier studies have included both primagravida and multigravida patients. In the latter group, the diagnosis of preeclampsia is particularly prone to error.

Chesley et al.[589] at the Margaret Hague Maternity Hospital, followed 270 survivors of eclampsia from 1931 through 1974. Renal function (ability to concentrate urine or urea clearance) was normal in 97%. Three percent had significant proteinuria. The incidence of recurrent

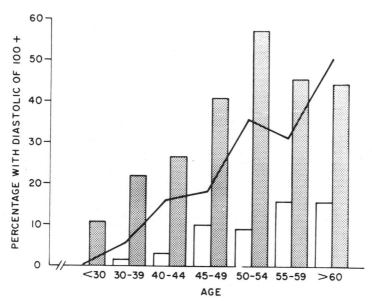

Fig 8–2.—Hypertension at follow-up in relation to age and the nature of pregnancies following eclampsia in nulliparas. *Solid line* represents women having had no later viable pregnancies; *open bars* represent women whose later pregnancies were all normotensive; *stippled bars* represent women who had at least one later hypertensive pregnancy. Each woman is represented by an average of 4.4 blood pressures recorded at intervals of about 7 years. (From Chesley L.C., et al.: The remote prognosis of eclamptic women. *Am. J. Obstet. Gynecol.* 124:446–459, 1976. Used by permission.)

eclampsia was 2.3%, and 19.5% developed hypertensive disorders during subsequent pregnancies (Fig 8–2).

In a review of the literature regarding the prevalence of hypertension among the survivors of preeclampsia-eclampsia, Chesley[589] found an average prevalence of 23.8% in 2,637 women, with various reviews reporting a prevalence ranging from 0% to 78%.

Chesley's[589] series contained 206 women who had eclampsia as multigravidas. Follow-up blood pressures were obtained through 1974 from 197 of the original 206 and compared with blood pressures obtained from four other studies of unselected women (Table 8–2). Using four different cutoff points of diastolic pressure, Chesley did not find a significantly greater frequency of chronic hypertension among patients who had had eclampsia one time, than among multigravidas. This supports the concept that pregnancy-induced hypertension does not lead invariably to chronic hypertension. The observations of

TABLE 8–2.—ACTUAL VERSUS EXPECTED PREVALENCE OF HYPERTENSION IN NONPREGNANT WOMEN WITH HISTORY OF ECLAMPSIA*

	DIASTOLIC PRESSURE (MM HG)			
	90+	94+	100+	104+
Actual number	94	56	46	23
Expected number				
Wetherby (1935)	100		52	
Gover (1948)	115		63	
Boe et al. (1957)	104		42	
Hamilton et al. (1954)	92		46	
Saller (1928)		65		29

*Modified from Chesley L.C., Annitto J.E., Cosgrove R.A.: *Am. J. Obstet. Gynecol.* 124:446, 1976.

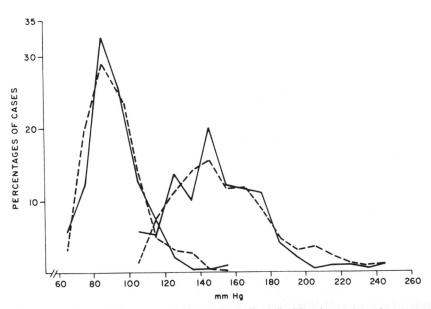

Fig 8–3.—The distribution of systolic and diastolic blood pressure in women who had eclampsia as nulliparas *(solid lines),* as compared with the distribution to be expected from the epidemiologic study of Hamilton and co-workers, 1954 *(broken lines).* (From Chesley L.C., et al.: The remote prognosis of eclamptic women. *Am. J. Obstet. Gynecol.* 124:446–459, 1976. Used by permission.)

Bryans[590] in another large series with long-term follow-up similarly supports this conclusion.

When Chesley's data[591] are displayed graphically in comparison with Hamilton's data[592] obtained from unselected women, no differences are seen between the distribution of the systolic or diastolic pressure of women who have had eclampsia as primagravidas and unselected women (Fig 8–3). In contrast, a similar comparison of blood pressure obtained from women who had eclampsia as multigravidas (Fig 8–4) show more hypertension among such women and unselected patients. Chesley interprets this observation as indicating that some of the women who had eclampsia as multigravidas may have had essential or renal parenchymal hypertension that predisposed them to develop eclampsia.

A more contemporary experience has been reported by Svensson, Andersch, and Hansson,[593] who collected data on 260 women with preeclampsia or hypertension during pregnancies occurring between 1969 and 1973. Reexaminations were carried out 7–12 years later in 237 patients, of whom 62 were found to have hypertension, defined as being under treatment or with blood pressure exceeding 160/100 mm

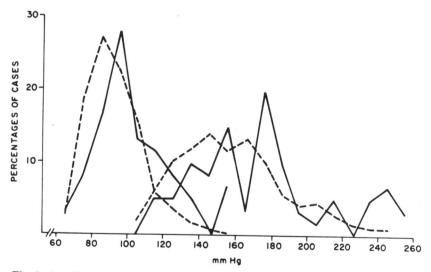

Fig 8–4.—The distributions of systolic and diastolic pressures in women who had eclampsia as multiparas *(solid lines)*, as compared with the distributions to be expected from the epidemiologic study of Hamilton and co-workers, 1954 *(broken lines)*. (From Chesley L.C., et al.: The remote prognosis of eclamptic women. *Am. J. Obstet. Gynecol.* 124:446–459, 1976. Used by permission.)

Hg, 24 had borderline hypertension, and 172 were normotensive. Those patients with antecedent hypertension were more likely to have severe preeclampsia and, along with those with severe gestational hypertension, more likely to have later hypertension than those with mild preeclampsia. Other factors that seemed to predispose to late hypertension were repeated hypertensive pregnancies and a positive family history of hypertension.

These data are consistent with those of Chesley et al.,[589] and support the contention that mild preeclampsia does not predispose to later hypertension but that a hypertensive diathesis, evidenced by preceding hypertension, a positive family history, repeated hypertensive pregnancies, and a history of severe superimposed preeclampsia, is indeed significant. Further, while those individuals who develop preeclampsia during a first pregnancy are no more likely to develop later essential hypertension than the general population, it may be that those who fail to develop pregnancy-induced hypertension are even less likely to develop hypertension than the general population.

CHAPTER 9

GOALS OF ANTIHYPERTENSIVE THERAPY

Efforts to control blood pressure of any cause during pregnancy should be made with several goals in mind[594] (Table 9–1). After reviewing currently available evidence regarding the treatment of hypertension during pregnancy, the Joint National Commission on Detection, Evaluation, and Management of Hypertension made the following recommendation in its 1984 report:

"Hypertension during pregnancy may represent the self-limited syndrome of preeclampsia (pregnancy-induced hypertension) or chronic (essential) hypertension. In either situation, treatment of hypertension is beneficial. In women with preeclampsia, antihypertensive therapy has improved fetal survival. There is no clear agreement on the therapy of choice, and each physician must decide on appropriate therapy for the individual patient. Adverse effects on fetal development must be a concern with any drug during pregnancy. However, there has been no evidence of teratogenicity when antihypertensive drugs have been given throughout pregnancy. Methyldopa has been used extensively in pregnant women, but recent clinical studies indicate that β-adrenergic blocking drugs are equally effective in controlling blood pressure and improving fetal survival. Because captopril has been demonstrated to increase fetal mortality in pregnant animals, it should probably be avoided during pregnancy."

A particular problem arises at the time of delivery. Blood pressure rises during uterine contractions at the time of delivery, constituting a threat to cardiovascular homeostasis in the inadequately treated hypertensive pregnant patient. Ueland and Hansen[595] have shown that systolic blood pressure tends to rise by about 20 mm Hg during each uter-

121

TABLE 9–1.—Antihypertensive Therapy During Pregnancy

Maternal Goals:
1. Prevention of accelerated hypertension and its complications
2. Prevention of superimposed preeclampsia
3. Prevention of premature atherosclerosis and its complications
Goals relative to the well-being of the fetus:
1. Reduction of fetal wastage
    a. Prevention of prematurity and neonatal death
    b. Prevention of spontaneous abortion and stillbirth
2. Avoidance of drugs with potentially harmful long-term effects

---

ine contraction in a normal subject. It is during this stage that the acute physical effects of further blood pressure elevation in the hypertensive patient are most threatening, e.g., dissecting aneurysm, intracerebral hemorrhage, and acute pulmonary edema.

CHAPTER 10

ANTIHYPERTENSIVE MANAGEMENT

GENERAL CONSIDERATIONS

The evaluation of the hypertensive patient begins with a medical history and physical examination with the goals of assessing target-organ damage and finding secondary causes of hypertension. An attempt is made to date the onset of the hypertensive process and to determine levels of blood pressure measured at various times during the patient's life. Questions are asked about prior therapy, response, and side effects. A search is made for historic or physical evidence of involvement of the brain, retina, heart, lungs, peripheral vasculature, or kidneys in the hypertensive process. Similarly, questions are asked and physical evidence sought for the presence of the most frequently encountered secondary forms of hypertension: renal parenchymal disease, renovascular disease, pheochromocytoma, primary aldosteronism, Cushing's syndrome, and aortic coarctation. Table 10–1 lists the minimal laboratory studies needed to evaluate an uncomplicated hypertensive patient. Table 10–2 outlines the steps necessary to pursue the diagnosis of a secondary form of hypertension when specific clues are uncovered by the medical history or physical examination. Appropriate modification must be made in this algorithm for pregnant patients to shield the developing fetus from the hazard of radiation.

Table 10–3 outlines the therapeutic steps recommended by the Joint National Committee on Detection, Evaluation, and Treatment of High Blood Pressure,[1] which describe the therapy that most hypertensive patients will be receiving when they become pregnant. The various

123

TABLE 10–1.—Initial Evaluation of the Hypertensive Patient*

Medical History
Physical Examination
Laboratory Studies:
1. To determine severity of vascular disease and possible cause of hypertension:
   Hemoglobin
   Hematocrit
   Complete urinalysis
   Serum potassium
   Serum creatinine
   ECG
2. To assess cardiovascular risk factors and provide baseline for following possible adverse effect of antihypertensive medications:
   Total cholesterol
   High density lipoprotein cholesterol
   Fasting plasma glucose
   Serum uric acid

*Modified from the Joint National Committee on Detection, Evaluation, and Treatment of High Blood Pressure: The 1984 Report of the Joint National Committee on Detection, Evaluation, and Treatment of High Blood Pressure. *Arch. Intern. Med.* 144:1045–1057, 1984.

TABLE 10–2.—Screening Tests For Most Common Forms
of Secondary Hypertension

DISORDER	PRIMARY SCREEN	DEFINITIVE SCREEN
Renal artery stenosis	Transvenous digital subtraction renal angiogram or rapid sequence IVP*	Renal arteriogram and renal vein renins
Renal parenchymal disease	Dipstick urinalysis, BUN or creatinine	Creatinine clearance, ultrasound, renal biopsy when indicated
Pheochromocytoma	Urine VMA†, metanephrines or catecholamines	Adrenal CAT scan or arteriograms
Primary aldosteronism	Serum potassium	PRA and Aldo‡ after Na+ restriction, adrenal vein sampling
Cushing's syndrome	Rapid, overnight dexamethasone suppression	Longer dexamethasone suppression test, adrenal arteriograms
Coarctation of aorta	Cuff BP§ in legs	Aortogram

*Intravenous pyelogram.
†Vanillylmandelic acid.
‡Plasma renin activity and aldosterone concentration.
§Blood pressure.

drugs that fit each step, and their usual dose ranges, are listed in Table 10–4. The adverse effects associated with each type of agent are given in Table 10–5.

CONSIDERATIONS DURING PREGNANCY

Chamberlain et al.[596] have recently surveyed the practices of 1,093 obstetricians in the management of pregnant women with preexisting hypertension and preeclampsia. The physicians queried used antihypertensive drugs frequently, especially methyldopa and diuretics, but used sedatives to treat patients with the least blood pressure elevation. Preeclampsia was usually treated with bed rest and sedation. The authors concluded, "there was considerable unanimity in the replies, even though most of the treatments and practices have not been validated by controlled trials and two thirds of the obstetricians gave the same answers to most of the questions."

TABLE 10–3.—STEPPED-CARE APPROACH TO DRUG THERAPY*

STEP	DRUG REGIMENS
1	Begin with less than a full dose of either a thiazide-type diuretic or a β-blocker;† proceed to full dose if necessary and desirable
2	If blood pressure (BP) control is not achieved, either add a small dose of an adrenergic-inhibiting agent‡ or a small dose of thiazide-type diuretic; proceed to full dose if necessary and desirable;§ additional substitutions may be made at this point‖
3	If BP control is not achieved, add a vasodilator, hydralazine hydrochloride, or *minoxidil* for resistant cases.
4	If BP control is not achieved, add guanethidine monosulfate

*From the Joint National Committee on Detection, Evaluation, and Treatment of High Blood Pressure, The 1984 Report of the Joint National Committee on Detection, Evaluation, and Treatment of High Blood Pressure. *Arch. Intern. Med.* 144:1045–1057, 1984. Used by permission; copyright 1984, American Medical Association.
†β-blockers include atenolol, metoprolol tartrate, nadolol, oxprenolol hydrochloride, pindolol, propranolol hydrochloride, and timolol maleate.
‡These include centrally acting adrenergic inhibitors (clonidine hydrochloride, guanabenz acetate, and methyldopa), peripherally acting adrenergic inhibitors (guanadrel sulfate and reserpine), and an α-1 adrenergic blocker (prazosin hydrochloride).
§A high percentage (70%–80%) of patients with mild hypertension will respond to the above regimen using steps 1 and 2.
‖An angiotensin-converting enzyme inhibitor may be substituted at steps 2 through 4 if side effects limit further use of other agents or if other agents are ineffective. Slow channel calcium-entry blockers (diltiazem hydrochloride, nifedipine, and verapamil hydrochloride) have not been approved for therapy in hypertension but may be acceptable as steps 2 or 3 drug.

TABLE 10–4.—ANTIHYPERTENSIVE AGENTS*

TYPE OF DRUG	DOSAGE RANGE† (MG/DAY)	
	Initial	Maximum‡
Diuretics		
Thiazides and related sulfonamide diuretics		
Bendroflumethiazide	2.5	5
Benzthiazide	25.0	50
Chlorothiazide sodium	250.0	500
Chlorthalidone	25.0	50
Cyclothiazide	1.0	2
Hydrochlorothiazide	25.0	50
Hydroflumethiazide	25.0	50
Indapamide	2.5	5
Methyclothiazide	2.5	5
Metolazone	2.5	5
Polythiazide	2.0	4
Quinethazone	50.0	100
Trichlormethiazide	2.0	4
Loop diuretics		
Bumetanide§	0.5	10‖
Ethacrynic acid	50.0	200‖
Furosemide	80.0	480‖
Potassium-sparing agents		
Amiloride hydrochloride	5.0	10
Spironolactone	50.0	100
Triamterene	50.0	100
Adrenergic Inhibitors		
β-Adrenergic blockers¶		
Atenolol	25.0	100
Metoprolol tartrate	50.0	300
Nadolol	20.0	120
Oxprenolol hydrochloride	160.0	480
Pindolol	20.0	60‖
Propranolol hydrochloride	40.0	480‖
Propranolol, long acting (LA)	80.0	480
Timolol maleate	20.0	60‖
Central-acting adrenergic inhibitors		
Clonidine hydrochloride	0.2	1.2‖
Guanabenz acetate	8.0	32‖
Methyldopa	500.0	2,000‖
Peripheral-acting adrenergic antagonists		
Guanadrel sulfate	10.0	150‖
Guanethidine monosulfate	10.0	300
Rauwolfia alkaloids		
Rauwolfia (whole root)	50.0	100
Reserpine	0.05	0.25

TABLE 10–4.—*Continued*

| TYPE OF DRUG | DOSAGE RANGE[†] (MG/DAY) | |
	Initial	Maximum[‡]
α 1-Adrenergic blocker		
Prazosin hydrochloride	1.0	20‖
Combined α and β adrenergic		
blockers		
Labetalol**	200.0	1,200
Vasodilators		
Hydralazine hydrochloride	50.0	300‖
Minoxidil	5.0	100‖
Angiotensin-converting Enzyme		
Inhibitors		
Captopril	37.5	150‖
Enalapril maleate**	10.0	40
Slow channel calcium-entry blocking		
agents§		
Diltiazem hydrochloride	120.0	240††
Nifedipine	30.0	180††
Verapamil hydrochloride	240.0	480††

*All drugs are listed by generic name. From the Joint National Committee on Detection, Evaluation, and Treatment of High Blood Pressure, The 1984 Report of the Joint National Committee on Detection, Evaluation, and Treatment of High Blood Pressure, *Arch. Intern. Med.* 144:1045–1057, 1984. Used by permission; copyright 1984, by the American Medical Association.

†The dosage range may differ slightly from recommended dosage in Physicians Desk Reference or package insert.

‡The maximum suggested dosage may be exceeded in resistant cases.

§This drug has not yet been approved by the Food and Drug Administration for treatment of hypertension.

‖This drug is usually given in divided doses twice daily.

¶Atenolol and metoprolol are cardioselective; oxprenolol and pindolol have partial agonist activity.

**This drug has not yet been approved by the FDA.

††This drug is usually given in divided doses three or four times daily.

Activity

Bed rest and sedation are widely recommended. Curet and Olson[597] have studied the effect of 4 hours of daily bed rest in the left lateral decubitus position in 66 patients with chronic hypertension. Therapy with hydralazine was added if diastolic pressure exceeded 110 mm Hg. Three perinatal deaths occurred and 38.8% developed superimposed preeclampsia. However, when compared with the outcome of previous pregnancies, the perinatal mortality rate was lowered from 16.8% to 8.8%. Mathews[598] compared the effects of bed rest and sedation with

TABLE 10–5.—ADVERSE DRUG EFFECTS*

DRUGS	SIDE EFFECTS	PRECAUTIONS AND SPECIAL CONSIDERATIONS
	Diuretics†	
Thiazides and related sulfonamides	Hypokalemia, hyperuricemia, glucose intolerance, hypercholesterolemia, hypertriglyceridemia, and sexual dysfunction	May be ineffective in renal failure; hypokalemia increases digitalis toxicity; and hyperuricemia may precipitate acute gout
Loop diuretics	Same as for thiazides	Effective in chronic renal failure; cautions regarding hypokalemia and hyperuricemia same as above; and hyponatremia may be found, especially in the elderly
Potassium-sparing agents	Hyperkalemia	Danger of hyperkalemia in patients with renal failure
Amiloride hydrochloride	Sexual dysfunction	. . .
Spironolactone	Gynecomastia, mastodynia, and sexual dysfunction	. . .
Triamterene	. . .	. . .
	Adrenergic Antagonists	
β-Adrenergic blockers‡	Bradycardia, fatigue, insomnia, bizarre dreams, sexual dysfunction, hypertriglyceridemia, decreased high-density lipoprotein cholesterol	Should not be used in patients with asthma, chronic obstructive pulmonary disease, congestive failure, heart block (greater than first degree), and sick sinus syndrome; use with caution in patients with diabetes and peripheral vascular disease
Central-acting adrenergic inhibitors	Drowsiness, dry mouth, fatigue, and sexual dysfunction	. . .
Clonidine hydrochloride	. . .	Rebound hypertension may occur with abrupt discontinuance
Guanabenz acetate	. . .	Same as for clonidine
Methyldopa	. . .	May cause liver damage and positive direct Coombs' test result

TABLE 10–5.—*Continued*

DRUGS	SIDE EFFECTS	PRECAUTIONS AND SPECIAL CONSIDERATIONS
Peripheral-acting adrenergic inhibitors	Sexual dysfunction and nasal congestion	. . .
Guanadrel sulfate	Orthostatic hypotension and diarrhea	Use cautiously with elderly patients because of orthostatic hypotension
Guanethidine monosulfate	Same as for guanadrel	Same as for guanadrel
Rauwolfia alkaloids	Lethargy	Contraindicated in patients with a history of mental depression; use with caution in patients with a history of peptic ulcer
Reserpine	Same as for *Rauwolfia* alkaloids	Same as for *Rauwolfia* alkaloids
α_1-Adrenergic blocker		
Prazosin hydrochloride	"First dose" syncope, orthostatic hypotension, weakness, and palpitations	Use cautiously in elderly patients because of orthostatic hypotension
Combined α- and β-adrenergic blockers		
Labetalol hydrochloride§	Asthma, nausea, fatigue, dizziness, and headache	Contraindicated in cardiac failure, chronic obstructive pulmonary disease, sick sinus syndrome, and heart block (greater than first degree); use with caution in patients with diabetes

Vasodilators

Vasodilators	Headache, tachycardia, and fluid retention	May precipitate angina in patients with coronary heart disease
Hydralazine hydrochloride	Positive antinuclear antibody (without other changes)	Lupus syndrome may occur (rare at recommended doses)
Minoxidil	Hypertrichosis, ascites (rare)	May cause or aggravate pleural and pericardial effusions

TABLE 10–5.—*Continued*

DRUGS	SIDE EFFECTS	PRECAUTIONS AND SPECIAL CONSIDERATIONS
Angiotensin-Converting Enzyme Inhibitors†		
Angiotensin-converting enzyme inhibitors	Rash and dysgeusia (rare at recommended doses)	Can cause reversible, acute renal failure in patients with bilateral renal arterial stenosis; neutropenia may occur in patients with autoimmune-collagen disorders; and proteinuria (rare at recommended doses)
Slow Channel Calcium-Entry Blocking Agents§		
Slow channel calcium-entry blocking agents§	Headache, hypotension, and dizziness	. . .
Diltiazem hydrochloride	Nausea	Use with caution in patients with congestive failure or heart block
Nifedipine	. . .	. . .
Verapamil hydrochloride	Flushing, edema, and constipation	Same as for diltiazem

*From the 1984 Report of the Joint National Committee on Detection, Evaluation, and Treatment of High Blood Pressure. *Arch. Intern. Med.* 144:1050, 1984. Used by permission; copyright 1984, American Medical Association.
†Sudden withdrawal of these drugs may be hazardous in patients with heart disease.
‡This drug has not yet been approved by the Food and Drug Administration (FDA).
§These drugs have not yet been approved by the FDA for the treatment of hypertension.

those of normal activity and nonsedation in the management of non-albuminuric hypertension in later pregnancy. He summarized, "135 patients took part in a randomized control trial designed to determine whether bed rest or sedation is of any general benefit to either the mother or the baby in pregnancies complicated by mild nonalbuminuric and nonsymptomatic hypertension after the 28th week. The results suggest that they are not." Despite Mathews'[598] negative conclusion, the studies of Curet and Olson[597] and others suggest that rest is beneficial. In addition, there are no studies which suggest that increased activity has a beneficial effect. Thus, at present there appears to be little reason to change the conventional practice of advising periods of rest for hypertensive gravidas.

However, most patients with preeclampsia do well with conservative management based on the concept that the only definitive therapy for preeclampsia is delivery. In this respect, the record of Pritchard and his group[599, 600] is impressive. Their patients were confined to an ambulatory, minimal-care facility for close observation if their blood pressure rose above 140/90. Diuretic agents were not used and a regular diet was allowed. Blood pressure, renal function, proteinuria, weight, and measurements of fetal condition were monitored. If diastolic pressures rose above 110 mm Hg, hydralazine was given to prevent maternal complications of hypertension. Magnesium sulfate was used for signs of central nervous system irritability. Delivery took place either when the fetus was mature, or when signs of fetal distress or growth retardation developed, or when the signs of preeclampsia worsened. No maternal mortality occurred in 154 consecutive cases of eclampsia, while most centers report a maternal mortality of 5%–10%. Pritchard[599] reported 3 perinatal deaths in a series of 346 patients with preeclampsia.

The Volume Problem: Implications for Therapy

A normal pregnancy is accompanied by substantial increases in both total body sodium and total body water. Several studies have shown that total body water increases by about 6–8 L.[601] The greater part, some 4–6 L, is found in the extracellular compartment. Blood volume begins to increase during the first trimester. The rate of increase becomes much greater during the second trimester. The increase during the third trimester is slight, and some investigators observe a slight fall near term.[602] An increase in both plasma and red blood cell volume comprises the increase in blood volume, which has been found to vary from 20% to 100%.[602] Plasma volume rises from the eighth week, reaches a peak between the 20th and 32nd week of pregnancy, and remains relatively constant with delivery. The magnitude of the increase appears to be related to the size of the fetus.[603] Six to 8 weeks after delivery, plasma volume usually returns to nonpregnant levels. Normally, sodium is retained as required by the increase in blood volume and by the size of the conceptus, totaling somewhere between 500 and 900 mEq.[601, 604] Water is retained at term in a slight excess which varies from 1 to 2 L in women without edema to 5 L in those with edema. Edema in itself is not a manifestation of underlying pathology, but has been found in 35% to 80% of healthy women with normal pregnancies.[588].

The sodium and water retention that accompanies a normal pregnancy is astonishing in view of the fact that glomerular filtration rate increases by about 50% during pregnancy.[605] It is estimated that about 30,000 mEq of sodium are filtered daily during a normal pregnancy, while only about 150 mEq are excreted.[601] Part of this increase is probably the result of increased progesterone levels during pregnancy.[606] Progesterone is a smooth muscle relaxant, which causes vasodilation and increased renal blood flow. Additionally, progesterone is an aldosterone antagonist.[607] These two properties contribute to enhanced natriuresis during pregnancy. To prevent volume depletion and circulatory failure, a number of compensatory mechanisms come into play, some of which may await discovery. Clearly, there must be a substantial increase in renal sodium reabsorption to meet the great increase in filtered sodium load. One factor acting to balance sodium losses during pregnancy is the renin-angiotensin-aldosterone system which becomes activated. During normal pregnancy, plasma renin substrate and renin concentration are increased, plasma renin activity is greater, and plasma aldosterone levels are higher.[27, 28] However, the sodium-retaining properties of aldosterone are limited when normal subjects are given excess mineralocorticoids, and renal escape occurs after about 400 mEq of sodium have been retained.[601] Rising estrogen levels may also play a role in sodium retention during pregnancy[608] through sodium-retaining properties and by stimulation of the renin-angiotensin system as a result of enhanced hepatic synthesis of renin substrate. Alteration of renal hemodynamics and/or renal tubular transport function[601] may also play a role.

Irregardless of the mechanisms which prevent sodium and volume depletion during pregnancy, the volume receptors of the gravid circulation come to recognize the volume-expanded state as physiologic. Dietary sodium restriction or sodium loading result in appropriate changes in plasma renin activity and aldosterone secretion.[609] Diuretic agents and upright posture stimulate aldosterone secretion in normal gravidas,[601, 611] while exogenous mineralocorticoids cause sodium retention and a fall in aldosterone secretion.[612, 613] The administration of heparinoid, which inhibits aldosterone secretion, is followed by negative sodium balance in pregnant women.[614] When heparinoid is withdrawn, aldosterone excretion returns to the high levels characteristic of a normal pregnancy.[614] Thus, the gravid patient responds to changing physiologic circumstances with appropriate increments or decrements of a resting aldosterone level that is elevated above that found in the nonpregnant state.

Tarazi et al.[60] have measured plasma volume in patients with hypertension of varying etiologies and have demonstrated that in the case of patients with renal parenchymal disease and impaired renal function, diastolic blood pressure is directly proportional to plasma volume. When volume is reduced, as by hemodialysis, pressure falls. In contrast, the volume status of patients with essential hypertension is determined in part by pressure diuresis. As blood pressure rose in such patients, their kidneys excreted intravascular volume in an attempt to lower pressure. Plasma volume is inversely related to diastolic blood pressure in patients with essential hypertension who do not have renal failure. Studies of patients with essential hypertension concurrent with pregnancy and of patients with preeclampsia showed results similar to those found in nonpregnant patients with essential hypertension: intravascular volume was reduced.

Although patients with preeclampsia have been found to retain sodium and water in excess of that retained by women with normal pregnancies, a considerable body of data has shown that blood volume is contracted in preeclamptic patients.[615] Investigators during this century have repeatedly demonstrated that the hematocrit and the specific gravity of plasma increase in patients with severe preeclampsia.[615] Blekta et al.[616] found that the red blood cell mass of patients who develop preeclampsia does not differ significantly from that of a normal gravida. However, several groups of investigators have found that plasma volume is reduced in patients with preeclampsia,[615] the decrease amounting to as much as 30%–40% of normal in patients with severe preeclampsia. Blekta et al.[616] were able to detect a reduction in whole-blood volume before the clinical manifestations of preeclampsia developed. Lang et al.[617] have studied blood rheology in 23 patients with eclampsia and 10 with intrauterine growth retardation and demonstrated significantly increased viscosity, at high shear rates, associated with increased hematocrit and fibrinogen levels.

Arias[618] measured the blood volume of 20 patients with chronic hypertension and pregnancy. He found that these patients, as a group, had lower blood volume than normal gravidas and delivered infants of lower weights. The hypertensive patients who delivered infants of appropriate size for gestational age had a greater degree of volume expansion during pregnancy than those who delivered undersize children or stillbirths. Those patients who did not increase their blood volume by 60 ml/kg or more were likely to deliver growth-retarded children.

Soffronoff and his colleagues[619] have measured plasma volume in 51 hypertensive and 35 normotensive gravidas. Although a large range and considerable overlap in plasma and blood volume determinations was noted, mean values in hypertensive gravidas were found to be significantly depressed compared to pregnant patients with normal blood pressure. Those hypertensive patients with plasma and blood volume determinations near those of normotensive patients were found to have a good maternal and fetal outcome. The lowest intravascular volumes were found in pregnancies which were subsequently complicated by severe hypertensive disease and evidence of uteroplacental insufficiency.

Gallery et al.[620] have followed the changes in plasma volume that take place during pregnancy in normal and hypertensive gravidas. In 40 initially normotensive patients who eventually developed hypertension during the third trimester, plasma volume was found to expand normally during the first two trimesters, followed by a significant contraction of plasma volume in the third trimester. The contraction of volume occurred before the development of elevated blood pressure in 29 of the 40 patients. In 30 patients with chronic hypertension and pregnancy, blood pressure was inversely related to plasma volume, while fetal growth was directly related to plasma volume.

Changes in colloid osmotic pressure have been described in patients with pregnancy-induced hypertension. In a study of 55 pregnancies, Benedetti and Carlson[621] found colloid osmotic pressure to be 22.0 mm Hg before and 17.2 mm Hg after delivery in 23 normal subjects, while lower values of 17.9 and 13.7 mm Hg, respectively, were found in 22 patients with preeclampsia. In contrast, Goodlin et al.[621a] found no differences between normal and hypertensive gravidas.

Diet

Limited activity and dietary sodium restriction are known to have an effect on the blood pressure of many patients with essential hypertension. Blood pressure usually falls during hospitalization, but the fall is more pronounced when salt is removed from the diet. The effect of sodium restriction during pregnancy has been examined in a number of studies. Robinson[622] studied 1,039 pregnant patients on a high-sodium diet and an equal number of patients on an ad lib diet. He noted fewer complications of pregnancy in the group with the highest salt intake; however, the incidence of preeclampsia among primiparas was unchanged by sodium loading. Zuspan and Bell[623] manipulated dietary sodium in preeclamptic subjects and concluded that the severity of the disease process determined how well the sodium was tolerated. Mengert and Tacchi[624] and Bower[625] also concluded that patients with mild preeclampsia tolerated sodium without difficulty.

In a recent uncontrolled study, Foote and Ludbrook[626] examined the effect of a 180-mEq sodium diet on the clinical course of 4 patients with essential hypertension and 7 patients with preeclampsia. The patients with preeclampsia did not worsen but there was not a noticeable improvement in their condition. Three of the 4 patients with essential hypertension responded to a high-salt diet with a fall in blood pressure and a rise in estriol excretion rates, suggesting improved placental perfusion. However, the lack of a suitable control group makes the effect of the added salt difficult to separate from the effects of rest, sedation, and careful observation. It is important to be mindful of the fact that individuals vary in their sensitivity to sodium and that patients with essential hypertension are more likely to develop an increase in blood pressure when sodium loaded than normotensive patients would. Therefore, it is unlikely that any study that involves an adequate number of patients will demonstrate a uniformly beneficial or detrimental response to sodium loads.

Diuretic Agents

The administration of thiazides is followed by diuresis and saluresis with an initial reduction in extracellular fluid volume, plasma volume, and cardiac output, and an increase in vascular resistance. Two or 3 months later, blood pressure remains reduced in 40%–50% of hypertensive patients, while plasma volume and cardiac output return towards pretreatment levels.[627, 628, 629] Thus, the long-term reduction of blood pressure is accompanied by a fall in peripheral vascular resistance.[630]

The decrease in resistance has been attributed to a loss of sodium and water from vascular smooth muscle, which reduces the degree of encroachment on the cross-sectional areas of the resistance arteriole and also reduces responsiveness to pressor agents.[631] However, it has

not been possible to demonstrate a normalization of the water or sodium content of the arterial walls of animals with experimental hypertension after diuretic treatment.[632, 633, 634] Tarazi et al.[635] have noted
that total body water remains reduced during chronic thiazide therapy.
Additionally, plasma renin activity ordinarily remains elevated during
thiazide administration and falls to control levels when thiazides are
withdrawn, suggesting that a degree of volume depletion persists during long-term administration of the thiazide diuretics.

The use of thiazide diuretics during pregnancy has undergone extensive study. Attitudes concerning their use have changed dramatically.
Initially, Finnerty treated 16 preeclamptic patients with diuretics and
noted that blood pressure and proteinuria improved.[636] However, Salerno and his co-workers[637] studied 24 patients with preeclampsia and
noted that the disease process appeared to worsen in 11 patients
treated with diuretics. MacGillivray[638] studied 8 patients with preeclampsia and noted that diuretics did not appear to change the disease process even though the edema improved, suggesting that diuretics treated the signs rather than the cause of the disease.

Finnerty and Bepko[639] later studied about 3,000 patients assigned alternatively to groups receiving either prophylactic thiazides or no therapy. A reduced incidence of preeclampsia and a lower perinatal mortality rate was noted in the group receiving diuretics. However, Kraus
and his colleagues[640] conducted a randomized, controlled study of 195
nulliparas who were placed on hydrochlorothiazide and 210 nulliparas
who were placed on placebo. The incidence of superimposed preeclampsia was 6.67% in both groups.

Lindheimer and Katz[601] have concluded, "it remains to be established if the increment in maternal extracellular volume is required for
optimal uteroplacental perfusion, but it is noteworthy that in two complications of gravidity, preeclampsia and essential hypertension, intravascular volume is decreased and placental perfusion compromised.
Relations between volume status and vascular reactivity need to be
clarified. If preeclamptic vasoconstriction is an overcompensation to intravascular volume contraction, sodium salts may well be therapeutic.
However, if as in certain experimental models, hypervolemia sensitizes
the vascular receptors to the effect of endogenous pressor amines or
peptides, excessive salt could be clearly harmful. To date, claims that
either salt loading or its restriction, with or without diuretic therapy,
reduces the incidence of preeclampsia are unconvincing when scruti-
nized critically."

Given the observation that the initiation of diuretic therapy causes a decrease in plasma volume, cardiac output, and the rise in vascular resistance, it is my practice to avoid *adding* thiazide diuretics to the antihypertensive program of pregnant patients, unless needed for the relief of pulmonary edema. Whether it is beneficial or harmful to *continue* diuretic agents as part of the therapeutic program of patients with chronic hypertension who become pregnant remains to be established. Under these circumstances, diuretics may be harmless, since chronic therapy is accompanied by a return of plasma volume and cardiac output to levels near those observed before treatment. Alternately, chronic thiazide therapy may hinder the physiologic expansion of plasma volume which is essential to the successful outcome of the pregnancy. Until this point is resolved, I believe it to be the safer course to manage essential hypertension without diuretic agents during pregnancy when it is possible to obtain satisfactory control of pressure with other antihypertensive agents (see Table 10–3).

Plasma Expansion

The other mode of therapy which has been used in attempts to correct the hemoconcentration, contracted intravascular volume, and proteinuria of pregnancy-induced hypertension is the intravenous infusion of noncrystalloid solutions such as dextran and human albumin. Over the past two decades, several authors have recommended this type of therapeutic intervention.[641, 642, 643, 644, 645, 646, 647] However, all published reports are of studies that include relatively few patients, are not randomized, and do not include suitable control groups treated concurrently. In a widely cited study, Cloeren et al.[645] studied 20 patients with preeclampsia. Eighteen were found to have a low central venous pressure, ranging from 0 to -7 cm H_2O, close to those of patients with severe burns or shock. The normal central venous pressure in the other patients was attributed to right heart failure. Fifteen patients received treatment with 6% salt-free Macrodex, 10% Rheomacrodex, or 20% low-salt human albumin, in volumes ranging from 100 to 2,500 ml, given over a few hours each day. All patients showed an increase in central venous pressure. The percentile of newborn size ranged from less than 5 to 95. Using indium-113-gelatin as a tracer, uteroplacental and uterine blood volumes were measured before and after volume expansion in 5 cases, all of whom showed an increase in uteroplacental blood volume. Diastolic blood pressure fell in the 8 patients who underwent continuous monitoring with an Arteriosonde but the magnitude of the reduction was not stated. Similar studies have been carried out by Brewer[641] and MacLean et al.,[647] with results suggesting that renal and placental perfusion were improved. Although this study suggests that preeclamptic patients with a low central venous pressure can receive cautious therapy with plasma expanders without ill effect, the lack of a suitable control group makes it difficult to assess the degree of benefit, if any, received by the patients. In addition, this study does not claim that all patients with preeclampsia or with pregnancies complicated by hypertension require therapy with plasma expanders.

Jouppila et al.[648] have studied the effect of albumin infusion on intervillous blood flow in 13 patients with severe preeclampsia, using intravenously administered [133]xenon to measure flow. Although serum albumin concentration and colloid osmotic pressure rose significantly, there was no improvement in intravillous blood flow, leading these investigators to question the value of using infusions of albumin to improve placental circulation in patients with severe preeclampsia.

Goodlin et al.[649] have measured plasma volume in 200 patients with various complications of pregnancy to determine if any simple clinical test allowed identification of the hypovolemic patient. They concluded that plasma volume must be measured directly, since no other routine laboratory measurement was predictive. They recommended that the expansion of intravascular volume in pregnant patients should be a major goal of antenatal care. As pointed out by Redman[650] in a recent editorial, this recommendation is based on the assumption that reduced plasma volume causes fetal growth retardation; however, since plasma volume has been shown to be directly related to the size of the conceptus, the reduced plasma volume found in some patients with preeclampsia might be the result, rather than the cause, of a growth-retarded fetus. Redman further notes that at present, a randomized controlled trial is needed to see if expansion of plasma volume has a beneficial effect on the outcome of pregnancy.

Thus, the pendulum has swung from the liberal use of diuretics during pregnancy to the use of liberal salt diet and plasma expanders. As once was the case with the use of diuretics, large, randomized, controlled studies with monitoring of pulmonary capillary wedge pressure and other hemodynamic variables are now needed to define the place of plasma expanders in the treatment of patients with hypertensive pregnancies. At present, I believe that specific indications such as hypotension should be present before deviating from Pritchard's[599] recommendation that hydration should be limited to crystalloid solution infused at a rate of 60–120 ml/hr. It must not be forgotten that arterial blood pressure is the product of total peripheral resistance and cardiac output. If cardiac output is increased by expansion of blood volume, without reduction of the total peripheral resistance, i.e., relieving the vasospasm of pregnancy-induced hypertension, blood pressure will show a further increase. If the increase in pressure is great enough, the patient will be subjected to the acute effects of severe hypertension, cerebral hemorrhage, acute pulmonary edema, and aortic dissection.

Centrally Acting and Other Agents Which Block the Sympathetic Nervous System

The antihypertensive agents with which internists and family practitioners are most familiar have received relatively little study in the management of hypertensive pregnancies. For example, clonidine and guanabenz, two agents which stimulate central nervous system α-2 receptors, thus reducing sympathetic outflow to the periphery, have not been used extensively to treat hypertensive patients during pregnancy, and the safety of doing so has not been established. At present, methyldopa, an agent with a similar mechanism of action, has received the widest investigation. Kincaid-Smith et al.[651] treated 32 patients with methyldopa and observed a perinatal loss of 9.3%, which was better than their predicted results, and a rate of development of preeclampsia of 38%, which was no better than predicted. Leather et al.[652] treated 22 patients with methyldopa and compared the results with 24 untreated patients. No fetal loss occurred in the 22 patients treated with methyldopa, and a fetal loss of 25% was seen in those not treated. Redman et al.[653] conducted a randomized study of 101 patients and 107 control subjects. The fetal salvage rate was slightly improved, largely because of fewer second-trimester abortions. No change was noted in the frequency of superimposed preeclampsia.

Studies of the disposition of methyldopa during pregnancy have shown that methyldopa crosses the placenta and that tissue levels in the fetus are equivalent to those of the mother. Ounsted et al.[654] have reviewed the development during the first 4 years of life of children born of hypertensive mothers, some of whom were treated with methyldopa. They found that maternal hypertension itself was associated with a slight developmental delay in childhood and that therapy with methyldopa during pregnancy did not worsen the delay and may even have reduced delay in neonatal development.

Reserpine, which prevents a reuptake of norepinephrine by nerve endings, is not used in pregnancy because it causes nasal obstruction in the newborn. Guanethidine and guanadrel, which work by interfering with impulse transmission by sympathetic ganglia, are seldom used in pregnancy because of postural hypotension.

β-Adrenergic Receptor Blocking Agents

Propranolol, widely used for the management of essential hypertension, has been used to treat small groups of patients with hypertensive pregnancies. Fetal growth retardation, neonatal bradycardia, and hypoglycemia have been reported. However, Eliahou et al.[655] treated 25 hypertensive, pregnant patients with propranolol and noted a reduction of predicted fetal wastage. Tcherdakoff et al.[656] studied 9 patients and noted good blood pressure control with no increase in fetal mortality. However, Lieberman and his colleagues[657] have recently treated 9 patients with hypertensive pregnancies and concluded that the probability of fetal neonatal death was increased by propranolol therapy. Pruyn et al.[658] followed 10 patients who received propranolol during hypertensive pregnancies, observed evidence of fetal growth retardation, but found no correlation with neonatal hypoglycemia, hyperbilirubinemia, apnea, or bradycardia. Sotalol,[659] metoprolol,[660] and labetalol,[661] the last a combined α- and β-blocker, have been used to treat small groups of hypertensive patients during pregnancy without notably dangerous side effects. Labetalol has been demonstrated to lower blood pressure without reducing uteroplacental blood flow measured by the indium 113 technique, suggesting that this agent decreases uteroplacental resistance.[662] Lamming and Symonds[663] treated 19 patients with pregnancy-induced hypertension with either labetalol or methyldopa and observed better blood pressure control and more frequent spontaneous labor in the group treated with labetalol. No adverse effects on the fetus were noted. Gallery et al.[664] randomly allocated 53 hypertensive gravidas to groups treated with either methyldopa or oxprenolol and concluded that the outcome of pregnancy, judged by greater maternal plasma volume expansion, placental growth, and fetal growth, was better in the group treated with oxprenolol. There was no evidence of harmful effect on the fetus; indeed, neonatal blood sugar concentration was higher in the children of mothers treated with oxprenolol.

Rubin et al.[665] compared atenolol, 100–200 mg daily, to placebo in a prospective, randomized double-blind trial which involved 120 women admitted to the hospital because of the development of hypertension during the third trimester of a previously normal pregnancy. Before treatment, blood pressure ranged between 140/90 to 170/110 mm Hg. Blood pressure was significantly reduced in the patients receiving atenolol, while pressures climbed to levels above 170/110 in one third of the patients treated with bed rest and placebo. Ten patients in the placebo group, but only 3 of the atenolol-treated group, developed significant proteinuria. Intrauterine growth retardation, neonatal hypoglycemia, and hyperbilirubinemia occurred equally in the two groups, while the symptoms of respiratory distress were seen in only 1 infant whose mother received placebo. Neonatal bradycardia was more common in infants of atenolol-treated mothers. These data indicate that atenolol effectively lowered blood pressure in patients with preeclampsia without worsening maternal or fetal outcome and may reduce the frequency with which proteinuria appears and hypertension accelerates.

Acute therapy with propranolol or β-adrenergic receptor blockers results in a fall in cardiac output and an elevation of peripheral vascular resistance. Lund-Johansen[666] has observed that these changes persist throughout 5 years of treatment. Thus, the hemodynamic effects of β-blockade might be expected to persist throughout pregnancy. Therefore, data exist on both sides of the issue, and the relative risk-benefit ratio of therapy with β-adrenergic receptor blockers during hypertensive pregnancies remains to be established definitely.

Vasodilators

Hydralazine is widely used in the treatment of hypertensive pregnancies, particularly through the intravenous or intramuscular routes, when blood pressure is substantially elevated. It is very effective parenterally, but as a long-term oral therapy, it is subject to several poorly tolerated side effects. Pregnancies are associated with a high cardiac output. Hydralazine, acting as a direct vasodilator and possibly as a cardiac stimulant, further increases cardiac output while reducing peripheral vascular resistance. Patients experience flushing, headache, tachycardia, and palpitations. Hydralazine may induce additional reductions in uteroplacental blood flow. Although Johnson and Clayton[667] found evidence that myometrial sodium 24 clearance increased after hydralazine, Gant et al.[668] have presented evidence that hydralazine causes a reduction in uterine blood flow. Using the indium 113 method to measure uteroplacental blood flow, Lunell et al.[669] recently found no reduction in uteroplacental blood flow after reduction of blood pressure in preeclamptic patients with intravenously administered dihydralazine. Vink et al.[670] have treated 33 hypertensive gravidas, whose diastolic blood pressure exceeded 110 mm Hg, with dihydralazine, monitoring fetal heart rate for evidence of reduced placental blood flow as arterial pressure was lowered. Fetal heart rate decreased in 19 pregnant subjects, 14 of whom delivered growth-retarded fetuses, while only 1 of 14 in whom fetal heart rate did not fall was retarded in growth, suggesting that a reduction in placental blood flow, if it occurs, presents a problem only in certain individuals. Many physicians now limit the use of hydralazine to situations in which severely elevated blood pressure must be controlled quickly and to a short period of time before delivery.

Bott-Kanner et al.[671] have studied combination therapy with propranolol and hydralazine in the management of essential hypertension in pregnancy. They found that 13 patients tolerated the regimen without difficulty, blood pressure remained below 140/90 in all cases, and none of the patients developed preeclampsia. However, there was 1 unexplained stillbirth and 2 cases of hypoglycemia. The combination did not appear to offer unique advantages.

Prazosin, which causes vasodilation by blocking peripheral vascular α-1 receptors has received little study in the management of hypertensive gravidas. Diazoxide is effective in the treatment of many hypertensive emergencies, but has the disadvantage of relaxing the uterine musculature, thus halting labor. It has been suggested that this agent must be administered intravenously and rapidly as a bolus of 300 mg because of rapid binding of plasma proteins. Recent studies show that diazoxide can be given intravenously in pulses of 75 mg every 10 minutes until blood pressure is controlled. Diazoxide can also be effective as a continuous intravenous infusion. Long-term use of diazoxide should be avoided because of sodium retention, hyperglycemia, and hyperuricemia.

Sodium nitroprusside is widely used by internists for the treatment of a variety of cardiovascular disorders but can cause cyanide toxicity in the fetus. This threat has limited the use of this potent agent in the treatment of hypertension during pregnancy. Minoxidil, a potent, direct-acting vasodilator, has not been studied in the management of hypertensive pregnancies and must be used with caution.

Thus, of the currently available antihypertensive agents, methyldopa has received the most widely documented study in the management of pregnant hypertensives, and the children born of mothers so treated have undergone the longest follow-up observation. The weight of currently available evidence suggests that methyldopa is relatively effective and relatively safe during pregnancy. Until comparable studies demonstrate another antihypertensive agent to be superior, it is my practice to use methyldopa as the agent of first choice. When methyldopa alone is not sufficiently effective, hydralazine is added. The favorable experience with atenolol in a relatively large group of patients with pregnancy-associated hypertension[665] suggests that this agent can be used as an alternative to methyldopa.

Angiotensin-Converting Enzyme Inhibitors

Several compounds which block various components of the renin-angiotensin system are available or under development but do not appear to be useful in the management of pregnancy-induced hypertension or hypertension accompanying pregnancy. As will be discussed later, Sullivan et al.[672] found that intravenously administered teprotide, an angiotensin converting enzyme inhibitor, had no effect on blood pressure in 5 patients with preeclampsia until substantial diuresis with reduction of plasma volume was induced by furosemide. Pipkin et al.[673] administered captopril, another converting enzyme to pregnant ewes and rabbits and observed an increase in perinatal mortality. Ferris and Weir[674] have administered captopril to pregnant rabbits, beginning at the 15th week of gestation. Fetal survival was only 14% in the treated animals, in contrast to 99% in controls, even though blood pressure did not differ between the two groups. In addition, they found that captopril was associated with a fall in uterine vein PGE_2 concentration. When animals are given indomethacin to block uterine synthesis of PGE_2,[468] uterine blood flow falls. In humans, aspirin administered during pregnancy has been associated with high fetal mortality in one study by Turner and Collins,[675] but not in another conducted by Shapiro et al.[676]

Given the lack of efficacy in preeclampsia and the potential for fetal harm demonstrated by animal studies, there appears to be little reason to use this class of compounds to manage hypertension during pregnancy unless future studies uncover compelling new evidence supporting their use.

Calcium Channel Blocking Agents

In the field of cardiovascular therapeutics, an important recent advance has been the introduction of the calcium channel blocking agents. These compounds inhibit the passage of calcium ions into the cell, resulting in a reduction in contractility and vasodilatation and, as the slow calcium current is required for activity of cardiac conducting tissue, a slower transmission of impulses across the atrioventricular node.[677] While the first of these agents has been used in Europe since 1962, and many are widely used outside the United States for the treatment of angina pectoris, coronary vasospasm, atrial tachyarrhythmia, and hypertension, they have not yet received approval for the latter use in the United States. The three compounds currently available in this country are nifedipine, verapamil, and diltiazem. Nifedipine is a potent vasodilator, useful for the treatment of vasospastic angina and for the rapid control of severe hypertension. Fluid retention accompanies chronic use of this compound. Verapamil lowers vascular resistance and also reduces myocardial contractility and atrioventricular conduction, thus the agent must be used with caution, or not at all, in patients with heart failure or disorders of cardiac conduction. The properties of diltiazem lie somewhere between those of nifedipine and verapamil.

These agents have not been investigated systematically relative to the management of essential hypertension during pregnancy, or of preeclampsia of varying degrees of severity, but have been used in individual patients with good results. However, as pointed out in a recent review by Zaret,[678] there is reason to speculate that the antivasospastic properties of these compounds might make them particularly useful in the treatment of preeclampsia, a consideration which is sufficiently attractive to warrant further study.

Progesterone Therapy

Sammour et al.[679] have used progesterone, 600 mg daily, to treat 15 patients with preeclampsia while following another 10 such patients under conventional treatment. They reported a significant fall in systolic and diastolic blood pressure, an increase in urine output, and a

TABLE 10–6.—ANTIHYPERTENSIVE AGENTS IN PREGNANCY

DRUG	PRECAUTIONS IN PREGNANCY
I. Diuretics:	
Furosemide	Maternal: Water and electrolyte depletion
	Newborn: Fetal abnormalities in experimental animals
Thiazide	Maternal: Electrolyte depletion, hypokalemia, gout,
Diuretics	hypoglycemia, thrombocytopenia, and
	hemorrhagic pancreatitis
	Newborn: Thrombocytopenia
II. Sympatholytic agents:	
Clonidine	Maternal: Drowsiness, dry mouth, rebound
	hypertension
	Newborn: Inadequate data
Guanethidine	Rarely used in pregnancy because of postural
	hypotension
Methyldopa	Maternal: Lethargy, fever, hepatitis, positive
	Coombs test, hemolytic anemia
Metoprolol	Maternal: Cardiac failure, bradycardia, bronchospasm if
	dose sufficient
	Newborn: Inadequate data
Prazosin	Maternal: First-dose syncope
	Newborn: Inadequate data
Propranolol	Maternal: Cardiac failure, bronchospasm, bradycardia
	Newborn: Growth retardation, hypoglycemia,
	bradycardia, apnea
Reserpine	Maternal: Depression, nasal stuffiness, extrapyramidal
	signs and increased sensitivities to seizures,
	peptic ulcer
	Newborn: Increased respiratory tract secretions, nasal
	congestion, cyanosis, and anorexia
III. Vasodilators:	
Hydralazine	Maternal: Flushing, headache, tachycardia, palpitations,
	angina pectoris, lupus syndrome
Minoxidil	Maternal: Fluid retention, hirsutism, tachycardia,
	pericardial effusion
	Newborn: Inadequate data
Sodium nitroprusside	Maternal: Hypotension
	Newborn: Cyanide toxicity
IV. Angiotensin converting	Maternal: Hypotension, neutropenia, renal failure,
enzyme inhibitors	proteinuria
	Newborn: Increased perinatal mortality

lessening of edema, but no change in proteinuria in the progesterone-treated group. While interesting, these findings are unconfirmed and at present should form the basis for further study, not for therapy.

Precautions in Pregnancy

The potential adverse effects for mother, developing fetus, and newborn are summarized in Table 10–6.

CHAPTER 11

PATHOPHYSIOLOGIC SUBDIVISIONS OF ESSENTIAL HYPERTENSION

MANY INVESTIGATORS have concluded that essential hypertension does not constitute a single entity but instead might be the final common manifestation of a number of pathophysiologic processes, each associated with a distinct disorder of different mechanisms of blood pressure regulation.[680] The subgroups of essential hypertension which have received the most attention are those based on differences in responsiveness of the renin-angiotensin-aldosterone system[681] (Fig 11–1). In other hypertensive patients, differences in hemodynamic status have been observed, e.g., certain young patients with hypertension have a high cardiac output.[49] The normal pregnancy is characterized by a high cardiac output. Lim and Walters[682] have studied the hemodynamics of mild hypertension in pregnancy and have found an increase in both heart rate and cardiac index in subjects with pregnancy-induced hypertension. However, Lees[683] found that some patients with pregnancy-induced hypertension had an increase in total peripheral resistance. Thus, the controversy which has existed since the reports of Hamilton[39] and Werko[684] 30 years ago continues.

Abnormalities of the extracellular fluid compartments have also been described, and one group of essential hypertensive patients with unusually elevated plasma volume has been found.[60] A fourth subdivision involves activity of the sympathetic nervous system. A subgroup of patients with high plasma norepinephrine levels has been described.[102, 103, 104] Hypertensive patients in these subgroups frequently respond optimally to specific forms of antihypertensive therapy directed toward correcting a given abnormality, e.g., patients with low plasma renin activity presumably have a volume-dependent form of blood pressure elevation and respond well to diuretics but poorly to propranolol. In contrast, patients with high plasma renin activity often show a good response to propranolol, which inhibits renin release and subsequent angiotension II formation, or to angiotensin-converting enzyme inhibitors, which interfere with the formation of angiotensin II.

Hypertensive pregnancies are associated with relatively low plasma renin activity.[419, 427, 449] Patients who later develop preeclampsia are known to display an increased sensitivity to the pressor effects of angiotensin II.[685] Sullivan et al.[672] have studied the effect of the parenteral angiotensin-converting inhibitor, teprotide, in the management of patients with preeclampsia whose blood pressure elevation persisted immediately after delivery. Using doses of teprotide known to prevent the pressor response to infusions of angiotensin I, these investigators were unable to lower blood pressure until the patients were volume depleted (Fig 11–2). The observation that inhibition of angiotensin-converting enzyme does not lower blood pressure in patients with preg-

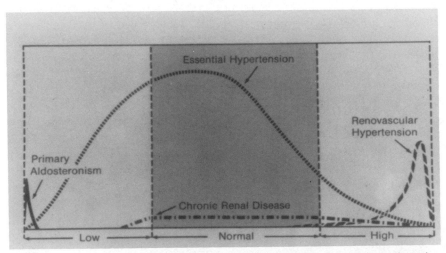

Fig 11–1.—Schematic representation of plasma renin activity in various hypertensive diseases. The expected number of patients with each type of hypertension is indicated along with their proportion of low, normal, or high renin levels. (From Kaplan N.M.: Renin profiles: The unfulfilled promises. *J.A.M.A.* 238:611, 1977. Used by permission; copyright 1977, American Medical Association.)

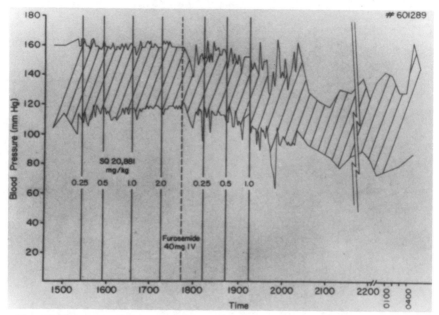

Fig 11–2.—Effect of angiotensin-converting enzyme blockade on arterial blood pressure 4 hours after delivery. *Vertical lines* denote intravenous dose levels of SQ 20,881 and furosemide and time of administration. Note lack of response until SQ 20,881 is administered after diuresis. Resting blood pressures without treatment on the day following the study are shown on the right-hand side of the figure. (From Sullivan J.M., et al.: SQ 20,881: Effect on eclamptic-preeclamptic women with postpartum hypertension. *Am. J. Obstet. Gynecol.* 131:707–715, 1978. Used by permission.)

nancy-induced hypertension[672] suggests that preeclampsia is a "low-renin" type of hypertension in which the elevation of blood pressure does not depend upon circulating angiotensin II levels, even though sensitivity to infused angiotensin II is enhanced. However, these findings do not eliminate the possibility that the renin-angiotensin system is involved in the initiation of the disorder.

Although pathophysiologic profiling of hypertensive subjects remains an interesting area for research,[680] there is at present no compelling evidence that such a characterization is of significant help in selecting therapy for patients with hypertensive pregnancies.

CHAPTER 12

MANAGEMENT OF PATIENTS WITH PREECLAMPSIA-ECLAMPSIA

THE MANAGEMENT OF patients with preeclampsia-eclampsia or pregnancy-induced hypertension has been the subject of a number of detailed reviews,[475, 476, 600, 686, 687, 688] as mentioned initially. One of the most difficult aspects appears to lie in making a correct clinical diagnosis. The definitive way to make a diagnosis is renal biopsy, but this is not a risk-free procedure and cannot be used frequently. The benefit of the information gained must be weighed against a high risk of hemorrhage.[689] However, in one study of 35 patients with a clinical diagnosis of preeclampsia, characteristic renal changes were found in only 26%.[387] These data suggest that improved methods are needed to make the diagnosis of preeclampsia without risking renal biopsy and suggest that the results of therapeutic trials are contaminated with patients who do not actually have preeclampsia-eclampsia but instead have chronic hypertension of various etiologies. Molar pregnancy or fetal hydrops are other diagnostic possibilities when signs of preeclampsia develop before the 24th week.

The preventive measures that have been proposed include careful observation to detect rapid weight gain or a tendency for the diastolic pressure to increase. Edema is an early sign, but it is not specific because it can also be seen in patients with normal pregnancies. Patients should be told to report persistent headache, visual disturbance, or swelling of the face or hands. Although widely prescribed, the restric-

151

tion of caloric or sodium intake has not incontestably demonstrated a beneficial effect, nor has sodium loading. Thiazide diuretics were used in the past to prevent preeclampsia, but a double-blind study has seriously questioned the value of this intervention.[640] Although there is some doubt that preeclampsia can be prevented, progression to eclampsia should be preventable by appropriate therapy. When a pregnant woman is near term, of course, either induction of labor or cesarean section will achieve such a goal.

When preeclampsia develops earlier in the pregnancy, hospitalization or strict bed rest at home is essential, and avoidance of sodium excess appears to be reasonable at this point, although many mildly preeclamptic patients can tolerate salt without difficulty.[622] Chesley advocates hospitalization if blood pressure exceeds 140/90, if a urine reaction for protein of 1+ or greater develops, or if weight repeatedly increases by 3 lb or more a week.[690] In the hospital, bed rest, close observation, and sedation are indicated. Such a regimen often results in spontaneous diuresis, loss of weight, and a fall in blood pressure; these changes began within the first 24 hours and blood pressure lowered to less than 140/90 by the fifth day in the series of Gilstrap et al.[691] When improvement takes place, the pregnancy can be continued with monitoring for fetal distress or growth retardation by sonogram and/or amniocentesis for the appearance of pulmonary stabilizing phosphorolipids indicating maturity. In the series of Gilstrap et al.[691] continued worsening of preeclampsia took place in 6% of patients, necessitating delivery.

As mentioned earlier, studies such as that of Gallery et al.[692] (in which 500 ml of a plasma protein solution was used to correct intravascular volume contraction in 14 patients with preeclampsia and a fall was noted in blood pressure in 12) have led to the practice of intravenously administering large volumes of fluids to patients with hypertension and pregnancy. Without adequate hemodynamic monitoring, this practice can lead to cerebral and pulmonary edema.

Severe preeclampsia is indicated by blood pressure elevation to levels above 160/110 and by irritability, increasing edema, and proteinuria. The consequences of severe preeclampsia to the mother are described in Table 12–1. Under these circumstances, therapy should be directed towards preventing the onset of convulsions that are associated with a major increase in fetal and maternal mortality. Ordinary measures include the use of parenteral magnesium sulfate, antihypertensive agents, osmotic diuresis with agents such as mannitol if oliguria is present, and prompt delivery to prevent progression to eclampsia and

TABLE 12–1.—Maternal Consequences of Severe Preeclampsia*

A. CNS complications
   1. Eclampsia
      a. Seizures
      b. Encephalopathy and coma
      c. Psychosis, self-limited
   2. Cerebral hemorrhage
B. Cardiopulmonary complications
   1. Pulmonary edema
      a. Usually noncardiogenic
      b. Left ventricular failure possible
      c. Potential for superimposed bacterial or aspiration pneumonia
   2. Pleural, pericardial effusions; ascites
   3. Cardiovascular collapse (shock)
      a. Rare complication within 24 hours postpartum
      b. Possible contributing role of diuretic therapy and unappreciated degree of hemorrhage, fluid loss
C. Renal disease (major manifestations)
   1. Acute renal failure
   2. Nephrotic syndrome
D. Abruptio placentae
E. Hematologic complications
   1. Thrombocytopenia
   2. Microangiopathic hemolysis
   3. Disseminated intravascular coagulation
F. Liver disease
   1. Mild functional abnormalities
   2. Subcapsular hemorrhage with pain (rare hepatic rupture)
G. Retinal detachment

*From Feinberg L.E.: Hypertension and Preeclampsia, in Abrams R.S., Wexler P. (eds.): *Medical Care of the Pregnant Patient*, Boston, Toronto, Little, Brown & Co., 1983, pp. 161–182. Used by permission.)

fetal death. Magnesium is given primarily to prevent seizures and in addition is a mild vasodilator. It is given intravenously as magnesium sulfate, 2–4 g of 10% or 23% solution, followed by a continuous infusion of 0.5–2.0 g/hr,[687] with adjustment made in the infusion rate so as to reduce hyperactive deep tendon reflexes to normal levels, without inducing respiratory depression or loss of reflexes, both signs of magnesium toxicity. If urine volume decreases, magnesium excretion becomes impaired and the rate of infusion must be reduced. Serum magnesium levels are a helpful guide to therapy. However, the lag time before results are available from many laboratories poses a problem. As pointed out by Feinberg[687] an intravenous infusion of 4 g given over 4 minutes results in a plasma concentration of 7–9 mEq/1. The therapeutic range is considered to lie between 4.8 and 8.4 mEq/1, loss of peripheral reflexes occurs at plasma levels above 10 mEq/1, respiratory muscle depression at levels above 10 mEq/1, and cardiac arrest at levels above 30 mEq/1. An intravenous infusion of 0.5–2.0 g/hr after a loading dose should produce levels of 4–7 mEq/1. Intramuscular administration offers an alternative, although less comfortable, route of administration and offers the advantage of requiring somewhat less frequent monitoring by hospital personnel than does the intravenous route.

Parenteral hydralazine is widely used when further reduction of blood pressure is necessary. Intravenously administered doses of 5–10 mg, given at 15-minute intervals until a diastolic pressure of 90–100 mm Hg is reached, should be followed by a constant infusion of 5 mg/hr, adjusted to maintain the diastolic pressure between 90 to 100 mm Hg. Prolonged infusions will result in compensatory fluid retention beyond that required to correct volume contractions accompanying preeclampsia and may necessitate the use of furosemide, 20 mg given intravenously, to potentiate the antihypertensive effects of hydralazine.

If convulsions or eclampsia develop in spite of therapy or, as more frequently happens, in the absence of prior therapy, a program should be initiated to prevent further convulsions, reduce vasospasm, lower blood pressure, and initiate diuresis. The appearance of convulsions is associated with loss of the fetus in as many as 25% of cases, and maternal mortality is as high as 25%. Causes of seizures other than eclampsia should be ruled out. The usual therapeutic measures in obstetrical practice include bed rest in quiet surroundings, with close observation and the use of parenteral magnesium sulfate with monitoring of serum levels, and parenteral hydralazine. The latter antihypertensive agent appears to have gained popularity since Assali presented evidence that drugs acting upon the autonomic nervous system are relatively ineffective in treating the vasospasm of patients with acute preeclampsia-eclampsia.[693] Recommended anticonvulsive therapy consists of 20 mg intravenously administered diazepam, 250 mg amobarbital, or 0.5–1.0 g phenytoin, while furosemide is given intravenously to promote diuresis.

When hydralazine does not control blood pressure adequately and delivery is planned within 30 minutes, intravenously administered sodium nitroprusside can be used to lower pressure more effectively. However, more prolonged use can result in fetal intoxication with cyanide. Sodium nitroprusside is both an arterial and venous dilator. Thus, this compound can be very effective in improving cardiac failure and pulmonary congestion due to acutely high arterial pressures and the fluid overload which can result from attempts to correct contraction of plasma volume. Use for such a purpose is best monitored with a

TABLE 12–2.—EVALUATION OF PATIENTS WITH PREECLAMPSIA/ECLAMPSIA*

PREECLAMPSIA (REMOTE FROM TERM)	PREECLAMPSIA/ECLAMPSIA (MATURE FETUS)
Thorough initial H & P† looking for signs and symptoms of severe preeclampsia	*Mild Preeclampsia* Thorough initial H & P† looking for signs and symptoms of severe preeclampsia Assess fetal maturity
Initial lab evaluation CBC‡ Urinalysis Serum creatinine, uric acid 24-hr urine protein, creatinine clearance, metanephrine	Fetal monitoring for signs of distress Initial lab evaluation CBC,‡ platelet count, urinalysis, serum creatinine, urine acid
Consider molar pregnancy if onset prior to wk 24	Serial maternal monitoring BP, weight, sensorium, fundoscopy, chest exam, reflexes, edema Intake and output
Assess fetal maturity via dates, uterine size, sonogram Serial fetal monitoring	Uterine protein CBC,‡ platelet count, uric acid
Serial maternal monitoring Daily review of symptoms Blood pressure Weight Fundoscopy Chest exam Reflexes Pelvic exam Urine protein 3 times/wk CBC‡ once weekly 24-hr urine protein and creatinine clearance 1–2 times/wk	*Severe Preeclampsia/Eclampsia* Intensive nursing care Initial lab evaluation Platelet count, blood smear, DIC§ screen, liver function tests, CBC,‡ urinalysis, chest roentgenogram, electrocardiogram Monitor MgSO₄ therapy: respirations, reflexes, urine output, seizures. Consider checking serum Mg+ + levels Consider Swan-Ganz catheter to monitor pulmonary capillary wedge pressure Workup seizures associated with focal signs, fever, stiff neck (i.e., electrolytes, glucose, CT scan, LP‖)

*Modified from Feinberg L.E.: Hypertension and Preeclampsia, in Abrams R.S., Wexler P. (eds.): *Medical Care of the Pregnant Patient,* Boston, Toronto, Little, Brown & Co., 1983, pp. 161–182.
†History and physical.
‡Complete blood count.
§Disseminated intravascular coagulation.
‖Lumbar puncture.

Swan-Ganz flow-directed pulmonary arterial catheter to allow measurement of left ventricular (pulmonary capillary wedge) filling pressures to guide titration of nitroprusside and furosemide.

Although controversy exists concerning the precise timing of delivery in the patient with eclampsia, there is general agreement that delivery should take place no later than at that point when the patient has stabilized under medical therapy. Some authorities advocate delivery as soon as the patient begins to respond to therapy.[694] The steps recommended in the management of patients with preeclampsia-eclampsia are summarized in Table 12–2.

CHAPTER 13

HYPERTENSIVE EMERGENCIES AND URGENCIES

THE DEVELOPMENT OF eclampsia is not the only hypertensive emergency that can complicate the course of a pregnant patient with high blood pressure. The other diagnostic possibilities that must be considered are outlined in Table 13–1. The clinical signs and symptoms associated with a hypertensive crisis are described in Table 13—2. Nine antihypertensive agents are available for parenteral use in the treatment of hypertensive emergencies and urgencies. Their dosages, onsets of action, and potential adverse effects are summarized in Table 13–3. It is my opinion that vasodilator drugs are the agents of choice in the treatment of hypertensive emergencies other than those associated with pheochromocytoma, where α-adrenergic receptor blockers are indi-

TABLE 13–1.—HYPERTENSIVE EMERGENCIES*

1. Malignant hypertension
2. Hypertensive retinopathy with fundal hemorrhages and symptomatic reduction in visual acuity
3. Hypertensive encephalopathy
4. Acute left heart failure due to hypertension
5. Dissecting aneurysm with hypertension
6. Subarachnoid hemorrhage with hypertension
7. Intracerebral hemorrhage with severe hypertension
8. Acute or advancing renal insufficiency with severe hypertension
9. Hypertensive crisis in pheochromocytoma
10. Eclampsia

*From Sullivan J.M.: Arterial hypertension, in Blacklow R.S. (ed.): *McBryde's Signs and Symptoms*, ed. 6. Philadelphia, J.B. Lippincott, Co., 1983, p. 288. Used by permission.

TABLE 13–2.—CLINICAL CHARACTERISTICS OF HYPERTENSIVE CRISIS*

Blood pressure: Usually >140 mm Hg diastolic
Funduscopic findings: Hemorrhages, exudates, papilledema
Neurologic status: Headache, confusion, somnolence, stupor, visual loss, focal deficits, seizures, coma
Cardiac findings: Prominent apical impulse, cardiac enlargement, congestive failure
Renal: Oliguria, azotemia
Gastrointestinal: Nausea, vomiting

*From Kaplan, N.M.: *Clinical Hypertension*, ed. 3. Baltimore, Williams & Wilkins Co., 1982, p. 198. Used by permission.

cated, dissecting aneurysm, where β-adrenergic receptor blockers are necessary, and perhaps subarachnoid or intracerebral hemorrhage, where vasodilatation might effect bleeding. The reason for this recommendation is the observation that most hypertensive emergencies are associated with marked elevation of total peripheral resistance, which falls, allowing cardiac output and organ perfusion to rise when vaso-

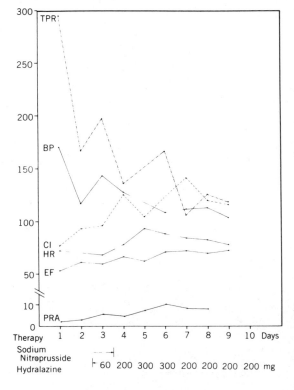

Fig 13–1.—Effect of vasodilator agents on hemodynamic variables and plasma renin activity (*PRA*, ng/mL/hr) in patient with severe hypertension. *TPR* indicates total peripheral resistance (dyne − sec − cm^{-5}) × 10^{-1}; *BP*, mean arterial blood pressure (mm Hg); *CI*, cardiac index (ml/ s); *HR*, heart rate (beats/ min); *EF*, ejection fraction (%). Note rise in PRA, CI, HR, and EF as TPR and BP fall. (From Sullivan J.M., et al.: Short-term therapy of severe hypertension. Hemodynamic correlates of the antihypertensive response in man. *Arch. Intern. Med.* 139:1233– 1239, 1979. Used by permission; copyright 1979, American Medical Association.)

TABLE 13-3.—DRUGS FOR MANAGING HYPERTENSIVE EMERGENCIES AND URGENCIES*

DRUGS	INTRAMUSCULAR DOSE, MG†	INTRAVENOUS (IV)		ONSET OF ACTION	ADVERSE DRUG EFFECTS
		SINGLE DOSE, MG	CONTINUOUS INFUSION‡		
Direct vasodilators Diazoxide		50–100 bolus§	15–30 mg/min over 20–30 min	3–5 min	Nausea, vomiting, hyperglycemia, hyperuricemia, hypotension, flushing, tachycardia, and chest pain
Sodium nitroprusside			50–100 mg/L	Instantaneous	Nausea, vomiting, muscle twitching, sweating, thiocyanate intoxication, and apprehension
Hydralazine hydrochloride	10–50	10–20||	200 mg/L	Intramuscularly 20–30 min; IV 10–12 min	Tachycardia, palpitations, flushing, headache, vomiting, and aggravation of angina
Nitroglycerine			0.5–10 µg/kg/min	2–5 min	Bradycardia, tachycardia, flushing, headache, vomiting, and methemoglobinemia
Sympathetic blocking agents Reserpine	1–5			2–3 hr	Drowsiness, stupor bradycardia, hypotension, and activation of peptic ulcer
Labetalol hydrochloride		20–80 IV bolus	2 mg/min	5–10 min	Vomiting, nausea, scalp tingling, burning in throat and groin, pain at injection site, postural hypotension, and dizziness
Methyldopate hydrochloride		250–500¶	1,000 mg/L	2–3 hr	Drowsiness
Trimethaphan camsylate			1,000 mg/L	5–10 min	Paresis of bowel and bladder, orthostatic hypotension, blurred vision, and dry mouth
α-Receptor blocking agents Phetolamine	5–15	5–15 (rapid injection essential)	200–400 mg/L	Instantaneous	Tachycardia and flushing

*From the Joint National Committee on Detection, Evaluation, and Treatment of High Blood Pressure: The 1984 Report of the Joint National Committee on Detection, Evaluation, and Treatment of High Blood Pressure. Arch. Intern. Med. 144:1045–1057, 1984. Used by permission; copyright 1984, by the American Medical Association.
†Start with the small dose shown. Subsequent doses and intervals of administration should be adjusted according to the response of blood pressure.
‡Start infusion slowly and adjust rate according to response of blood pressure. Constant surveillance is mandatory. Concentration of solution can be adjusted according to patient's fluid requirements.
§To be given at intervals of 5–10 minutes.
||The total dosage should be contained in a volume of at least 20 ml, and the solution should be administered from a 20- or 50-ml syringe. Blood pressure should be monitored continuously while the injection is being made. Rate of injection should not exceed 0.5 ml/min. To avoid hypotension, the injection should be stopped frequently when the blood pressure is falling.
¶Diluted up to 100 ml and injected during a 30- to 60-minute period.

Fig 13–2.—Combined sympatholytic-diuretic therapy of patient with severe hypertension. Reductions of blood pressure *(BP)* is accompanied by fall in cardiac index *(CI)*, which was elevated initially, while total peripheral resistance *(TPR)* actually rises. Pretreatment CI was normal in this group, but also fell after initiation of therapy. *HR* indicates heart rate (beats/min); *EF*, ejection fraction (%); *PRA*, plasma renin activity (ng/ml/hr). (From Sullivan J.M., et al.: Short-term therapy of severe hypertension. Hemodynamic correlates of the antihypertensive response in man. *Arch. Intern. Med.* 139:1233–1239, 1979. Used by permission; copyright 1979, American Medical Association.)

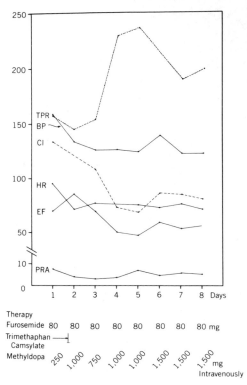

dilators are administered (Fig 13–1). In contrast, agents, other than peripheral α-receptor blockers, that interface with the activity of the sympathetic nervous system can reduce cardiac output, which, in the presence of diuretic-induced volume depletion, can cause compensatory vasoconstriction and potentially further impair organ perfusion (Fig 13–2).

CHAPTER 14

PREGNANCY AND SECONDARY HYPERTENSION

IN GENERAL, the younger the patient with hypertension, the more likely that patient is to have a secondary cause of hypertension. Since most women of childbearing age are relatively young, the possibility of an underlying cause of hypertension should be kept in mind. The most common cause of secondary hypertension in pregnant subjects is probably parenchymal renal disease; the most dangerous is pheochromocytoma.

HYPERTENSION SECONDARY TO RENAL DISEASE

Unilateral renal vascular disease has been estimated to be an etiologic factor in 5%–10% of the cases of severe hypertension occurring during pregnancy.[695] Severe hypertension has been reproduced in pregnant dogs and rabbits by renal artery constriction,[696] although under certain circumstances, blood pressure may be unaffected or even lowered by this intervention.[697, 698] Definitive diagnosis is made by renal arteriography and renal vein renin determinations, which should be considered in the postpartum evaluation of patients with an intravenous pyelogram showing differences in renal size or function, persistent, accelerating hypertension, or recurrent severe hypertension during successive pregnancies.

161

A number of renal parenchymal diseases have been associated with hypertension during pregnancy. These are acute and chronic pyelonephritis, acute and chronic glomerulonephritis, the nephrotic syndrome, polycystic kidney disease, diabetes mellitus with diabetic nephropathy, lupus erythematosus, scleroderma, periarteritis nodosa with renal involvement, and acute renal failure of various causes. The extensive literature relating to this subject has been reviewed by Schewitz[699] and by Sims.[370]

HYPERTENSION SECONDARY TO ADRENAL DISEASE

Pheochromocytoma is a rare cause of hypertension in nonpregnant as well as pregnant patients, but it is associated with a high maternal mortality rate when not discovered and treated.[700] Hendee cites 82 cases with a maternal mortality rate of 50% in undiagnosed patients, whereas only 1 of 11 patients in whom the diagnosis was made early in pregnancy died.[701] Pregnancy amplifies the symptoms of pheochromocytoma, and a clinical state resembling eclampsia can occur secondary to pheochromocytoma.

Primary aldosteronism is also a rare cause of hypertension in pregnancy that must be carefully differentiated from the state of secondary aldosteronism that occurs during normal pregnancy.[702] A case of severe hypertension during pregnancy secondary to an adrenal adenoma has been reported that was characterized by weakness and polyuria worsened by the administration of thiazide diuretics.[703] Cushing's disease has also been described as an unusual cause of hypertension during pregnancy.[704]

OTHER CAUSES OF HYPERTENSION IN PREGNANCY

Although coarctation of the aorta is frequently associated with blood pressure elevation above the area of constriction, this condition does not appear to be associated with preeclampsia.[705] The opposite appears to be the case with congenital hypoplasia of the aorta, which has been reported to cause cases of severe preeclampsia.[706, 707] Diabetes mellitus without apparent renal involvement[708] and erythroblastosis fetalis[709, 710] have been suggested as associated factors in some cases of preeclampsia-eclampsia.

LATE OR "TRANSIENT" HYPERTENSION

During uncomplicated pregnancies, peripheral vascular resistance increases at the end of gestation, giving rise to a blood pressure elevation of 10–15 mm Hg.[711] Certain individuals exceed this level during successive pregnancies but return to normal levels of blood pressure within 10 days of delivery. This clinical picture has been designated "late" or "transient", hypertension by the American College of Obstetrics and Gynecology. While the etiology of this condition is not understood; it has been proposed that elevated estrogen levels play a role, as they might in those patients who develop hypertension while taking oral-contraceptive agents.[419] Alternatively, patients with late or transient hypertension may be demonstrating the labile phase of blood pressure elevation that may precede fixed essential hypertension.[712] Because such patients may develop fixed blood pressure elevation in later life, regular measurement of their blood pressure is advisable.

CHAPTER 15

OPTIMAL BLOOD PRESSURE CONTROL

CONTROVERSY EXISTS about the degree to which elevated blood pressure should be lowered in patients with essential hypertension with concurrent pregnancy and in patients with pregnancy-induced hypertension. The dispute will be difficult to resolve until it has been established whether or not the uterine blood flow of humans undergoes autoregulation. In the pregnant ewe, it has been shown that uteroplacental blood flow is directly dependent upon arterial pressure, suggesting that this vascular bed does not autoregulate; therefore, lowering blood pressure reduces uteroplacental blood flow in this species[713] (Fig 15–1, 15–2). In contrast, the uteroplacental blood flow of the pregnant rabbit has been found to remain constant over a range of mean arterial perfusion pressure of 60–140 mm Hg[714] (Figure 15–3). The relevance of either experiment, which used healthy animals without hypertension or preeclampsia, to the problem of human essential hypertension or preeclampsia, remains questionable. Gant and his colleagues[668] have demonstrated that both chronic therapy with thiazide diuretics and acute therapy with either hydralazine or furosemide reduce the metabolic clearance rate of dehydroisoandrosterone sulfate in hypertensive gravidas (Table 15–1). If this measurement accurately reflects changes in uteroplacental blood flow under the clinical circumstances in which it was used, it implies that therapy with these particular drugs might be harmful to the fetus while nonetheless protecting the maternal circulatory tree. However, more recent studies which have used indium 113 to measure uteroplacental flow show that blood pressure can be lowered with agents such as dihydralazine[699] and labetalol[662] without a drop in placental perfusion.

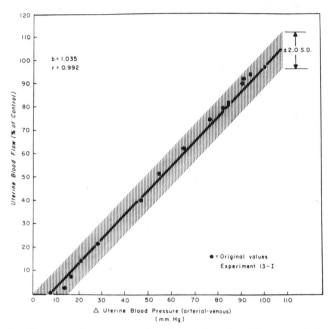

Fig 15–1.—Pressure-flow regression line determined from pooled proportionate data in term pregnant ewes. Since the relation is linear, uterine blood flow will vary with and in proportion to any change in perfusion pressure. (From Greiss F.C.J.: *Am. J. Obstet. Gynecol.* 96:41, 1966. Used by permission.)

Acting in accord with the concept that diastolic blood pressure of 109 mm Hg or less will not damage the maternal vascular tree if sustained for only a limited period, Pritchard[599] limited the use of antihypertensive agents to patients whose diastolic pressure exceeded 110 mm Hg, in which case hydralazine was given intravenously to prevent the adverse effects of acute severe hypertension. This conservative approach has been applied to 154 consecutive cases without a maternal death.

Nonetheless, several studies have shown that blood pressure elevation is associated with an adverse outcome of pregnancy. In many studies, antihypertensive therapy has not been shown to reduce the subsequent development of preeclampsia, but it does appear to reduce fetal wastage and probably prevents the development of short-term complications of hypertension: congestive heart failure, intracerebral hemorrhage, and dissecting aneurysm. More recent studies have shown that antihypertensive therapy prevents an increase in severity of essential hypertension and decreases the incidence of proteinuria during pregnancy, even though there was often no improvement in fetal outcome.[665, 715, 716] Therefore, it is my practice to maintain blood pressure at levels beneath 140/90 mm Hg when possible. However, clinical studies in this area involve small numbers and are not yet definitive. Continuation of effective antihypertensive therapy during pregnancy plays a part in preventing the long-term development of accelerated atherosclerosis. However, this goal could be deferred for 40 weeks if antihypertensive therapy were found to have an adverse effect on the outcome of pregnancy. Severely elevated blood pressure, i.e., diastolic levels above 110 mm Hg, definitely should not go untreated, since the hypertension might undergo further acceleration, and the patient might die of intracerebral hemorrhage, which is the most common cause of death in hypertensive pregnant women.[717] How mild a degree of blood pressure elevation requires or benefits from treatment has not been established. Adequately sized, randomized, controlled trials of the effect of various antihypertensive programs on the maternal and

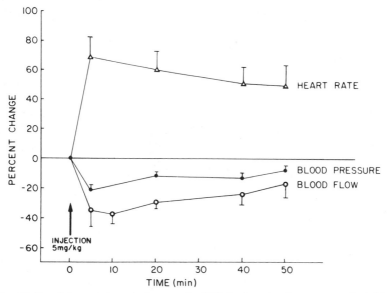

Fig 15–2.—Mean percent change (±SE) in heart rate, mean arterial blood pressure, and blood flow in the main uterine artery supplying the pregnant horn after bolus intravenous injection of diazoxide (5 mg/kg). The percent fall in uterine artery flow was about double the percent fall in blood pressure. All values were statistically significant ($P < .05$), $n = 7$. (From Caritis S.N., et al.: The effect of diazoxide on uterine blood flow in pregnant sheep. *Obstet. Gynecol.* 48:464–468, 1976. Used by permission.)

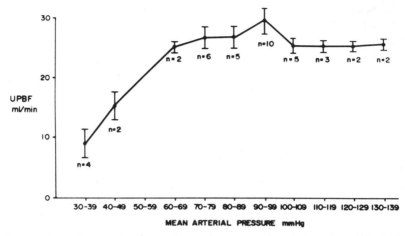

Fig 15–3.—The effect of varying perfusion on the uterine blood flow of the pregnant rabbit. Arterial pressure was raised by carotid ligation and lowered with antihypertensive drugs. Note the constancy of uterine blood flow over a range of mean arterial pressures, from 60–69 mm Hg to 130–139 mm Hg (*n*, number of observations at each arterial pressure). (From Venuto R. et al.: *J. Clin. Invest.* 57:938, 1976. Used by permission.)

fetal complications of pregnancies, trials in which patients are categorized by etiology and by different degrees of blood pressure elevation, are urgently needed to determine whether the reported changes in uteroplacental blood flow associated with the use of various agents has any clinical meaning, and under what circumstances antihypertensive treatment improves maternal and fetal outcome.

TABLE 15–1.—The Metabolic Clearance Rate of Dehydroisoandrosterone Sulfate (MCR-DS) and the Apparent Volume of Distribution (AVD-DS) Before and After Hydrochlorothiazide Administration[*]

PATIENT	CLINICAL CONDITION	MCR DS (L/24 hr)			AVD-DS (ml)		
		BEFORE	AFTER	%	BEFORE	AFTER	%
JII	Preeclampsia	52.6	37.9	28	8196	1666	79.6
RB	Chronic hypertension	165.4	52.0	70	13,888	7692	44.6
VJ	Excessive weight gain	46	22.4	51	8000	6536	18.3

[*]From Shoemaker E.S., et al.: The effect of thiazide diuretics on placental function. *Tex. Med.* 69:109–115, 1973. Used by permission.

REFERENCES

1. The Joint National Committee on Detection, Evaluation and Treatment of High Blood Pressure. The 1984 Report of the Joint National Committee on Detection, Evaluation and Treatment of High Blood Pressure. *Arch. Intern. Med.* 144:1045–1057, 1984.
2. 1984 Heart Facts Reference Sheet. Communications Division, American Heart Association, Dallas, Texas.
3. Rowland M., Roberts J.: Blood pressure levels in persons 6–74 years. United States, 1976–80. Advance Data. National Center for Health Statistics #84. U.S. Dept. of Health & Human Services, PHS Oct. 8, 1982.
4. Stamler J., Stamler R., Riedlinger W.F., et al.: Hypertension screening of one million Americans. *J.A.M.A.* 235:2299–2306, 1976.
5. Chesley L.C.: *Hypertensive Disorders in Pregnancy.* New York, Appleton-Century-Crofts, 1978.
6. Browne F.J.: Chronic hypertension and pregnancy. *Br. Med. J.* 2:283–287, 1947.
7. Wellen I.: The infant mortality in specific hypertensive disease of pregnancy and in essential hypertension. *Amer. J. Obstet. Gynecol.* 66:36–45, 1953.
8. Schewitz L.J., Friedman I.A., Pollak V.E.: Bleeding after renal biopsy in pregnancy. *Obstet. Gynecol.* 26:295–304, 1965.
9. Pollack V.E., Neettles J.B.: The kidney in toxemia of pregnancy: A clinical and pathological study based on renal biopsies. *Medicine* 39:469–526, 1960.
10. McCartney C.P.: Toxemia of pregnancy: A classification. *Clin. Obstet. Gynecol.* 9:864–870, 1966.
11. Rushmer R.F.: *Structure and Function of the Cardiovascular System.* Philadelphia, W.B. Saunders Co., 1972.
12. Mellander S., Johannsson B.: Control of resistance, exchange and capacitance function of the peripheral circulation. *Pharmacol. Res.* 20:117–196, 1968.
13. Bayliss W.M.: On the local reaction of the arterial wall to changes of internal pressure. *J. Physiol.* 28:220–231, 1902.
14. Folkow B., Neil E.: *Circulation.* New York, Oxford University Press, 1971.
15. Metcalfe J., Parer J.T.: Cardiovascular changes during pregnancy in ewes. *Am. J. Physiol.* 210:821–825, 1966.
16. Ueland K., Parer J.T.: The effect of estrogens on the cardiovascular system of the ewe. *Am. J. Obstet. Gynecol.* 96:400–406, 1966.
17. Bryant E.E., Douglas, B.H., Ashburn A.D.: Circulatory changes following prolactin administration. *Am. J. Obstet. Gynecol.* 115:53–57, 1973.
18. Chesley L.C.: Renal functional changes in normal pregnancy. *Clin. Obstet. Gynecol.* 3:349–363, 1960.
19. Metcalfe J., Ueland K.: Maternal cardiovascular adjustments to pregnancy. *Progr. Cardiovasc. Dis.* 16:363–374, 1974.
20. Herbert C.M., Banner E.A., Wakim K.G.: Variations in the peripheral circulation during pregnancy. *Am. J. Obstet. Gynecol.* 76:742–745, 1958.
21. McCall M.L.: Cerebral blood flow and metabolism in toxemias of pregnancy. *Surg. Gynecol. Obstet.* 89:715–721, 1949.

22. McCall M.L.: Cerebral circulation and metabolism in toxemia of pregnancy. Observations on the effects of veratrum viride and apresoline (1-hydrazinophthalazine). *Am. J. Obstet. Gynecol.* 66:1015–1030, 1953.
23. Pritchard J.A.: Changes in blood volume during pregnancy and delivery. *Anesthesiology* 26:393–399.
24. Hytten F.E., Paintin D.B.: Increase in plasma volume during normal pregnancy. *J. Obstet. Gynecol. Br. Commonw.* 70:402–407, 1963.
25. Pritchard J.A.: Hematologic aspects of pregnancy. *Clin. Obstet. Gynecol.* 3:378–385, 1960.
26. Rovinsky J.J., Jaffin H.: Cardiovascular hemodynamics in pregnancy. I. Blood and plasma volumes in multiple pregnancy. *Am. J. Obstet. Gynecol.* 93:1–15, 1965.
27. MacGillivray I., Buchanan T.J.: Total exchangeable sodium and potassium in nonpregnant women and in normal and preeclamptic pregnancy. *Lancet* 2:1090–1093, 1958.
28. Seitchik J.: Total body water and total body density of pregnant women. *Obstet. Gynecol.* 29:155–166, 1967.
29. Gray M.J., Munro A.B., Sims E.A.H., et al.: Regulation of sodium and total body water metabolism in pregnancy. *Am. J. Obstet. Gynecol.* 89:760–765, 1964.
30. Hytten F.E., Thomson A.M., Taggart N.: Total body water in normal pregnancy. *J. Obstet. Gynaecol. Br. Commonw.* 73:553–561, 1966.
31. Dexter L., Weiss S.: *Preeclamptic and Eclamptic Toxemia of Pregnancy.* Baltimore, Williams & Wilkins Co., 1941.
32. Thomson A.M., Hytten F.E., Billewicz W.Z.: The epidemiology of oedema during pregnancy. *J. Obstet. Gynaecol. Br. Commonw.* 74:1–10, 1967.
33. Adams J.Q.: Cardiovascular physiology in normal pregnancy: studies with the dye dilution technique. *Am. J. Obstet. Gynecol.* 67:741–759, 1954.
34. Assai N.S., Douglass R.A. Jr., Baird W.W., et al.: Measurement of uterine blood flow and uterine metabolism. IV. Results in normal pregnancy. *Am. J. Obstet. Gynecol.* 66:248–253, 1953.
35. Metcalfe J., Romney S.L., Ramsey L.H., et al.: Estimation of uterine blood flow in normal human pregnancy at term. *J. Clin. Invest.* 34:1632–1638, 1955.
36. De Swiet M.: The cardiovascular system, in Hytten F.E., Chamberlain G.V.P. (eds.): *Clinical Physiology in Obstetrics.* Oxford, Blackwell, 1980, pp. 3–42.
37. Szekeley P., Snaith L.: *Heart Disease and Pregnancy.* Edinburgh and London, Churchill Livingstone, Inc., 1974.
38. Burwell C.S., Strayhorn W.D., Flickinger D., et al.: Circulation during pregnancy. *Arch. Intern. Med.* 62:979–1003, 1938.
39. Hamilton H.F.H.: The cardiac output in normal pregnancy as determined by the Cournand right heart catheterization technique. *J. Obstet. Gynaecol. Br. Emp.* 56:548–552, 1949.
40. Ueland K., Novy M.J., Peterson E.N., et al.: Maternal cardiovascular dynamics. IV. The influence of gestational age on the maternal cardiovascular response to posture and exercise. *Am. J. Obstet. Gynecol.* 104:856–864, 1969.
41. Scott D.B., Kerr J.G.: Inferior vena caval pressure in late pregnancy. *J. Obstet. Gynecol. Br. Commonw.* 70:1044–1049, 1963.

42. Kerr M.G.: The mechanical effects of gravid uterus in late pregnancy. *J. Obstet. Gynecol. Br. Commonw.* 72:513–529, 1965.
43. Metcalf J., Ueland K.: The heart and pregnancy, in Hurst J.W., Logue R.B. (eds.): *The Heart* ed. 2. New York, McGraw-Hill Book Co., 1966.
44. Bader M.E., Bader R.A.: Cardiovascular hemodynamics in pregnancy and labor. *Clin. Obstet. Gynecol.* 11:924–939, 1968.
45. Ueland K., Hansen J.M.: Maternal cardiovascular dynamics. II. Posture and uterine contractions. *Am. J. Obstet. Gynecol.* 103:1–7, 1969.
46. Adams J.Q.: Cardiovascular physiology in normal pregnancy. Studies with the dye dilution technique. *Am. J. Obstet. Gynecol.* 67:741–759, 1954.
47. Frohlich E.D.: Hemodynamics of hypertension, in Genest J., Koiw E., Kuchel O., (eds.): *Hypertension.* New York, McGraw-Hill Book Co., 1977, pp. 15–49.
48. Widimsky J., Fejfarova M.D., Fejfar A.: Changes of cardiac output in hypertensive disease. *Cardiologia* 31:381–389, 1957.
49. Eich R.J., Peters R.J., Cuddy R.P., et al.: Hemodynamics in labile hypertension. *Am. Heart J.* 63:188–195, 1962.
50. Julius S., Randall O.S., Esler M.D., et al.: Altered cardiac responsiveness and regulation in the normal cardiac output type of borderline hypertension. *Circ. Res.* 36(Suppl. 1):I199–I207, 1975.
51. Ulrych M., Frohlich E.D., Dustan H.P., et al.: Cardiac output and distribution of blood volume in central and peripheral circulations in hypertensive and normotensive man. *Br. Heart J.* 31:570–574, 1969.
52. Julius S., Pascual A.V., Sannerstedt R., et al.: Relationship between cardiac output and peripheral resistance in borderline hypertension. *Circulation* 43:382–390, 1971.
53. Sannerstedt R.: Hemodynamic response to exercise in patients with arterial hypertension. *Acta Med. Scand.* 180(Suppl. 458):1–13, 1966.
54. Takeshita A., Mark A.L.: Decreased vasodilator capacity of forearm resistance vessels in borderline hypertension. *Hypertension* 2:610–616, 1980.
55. Al-Aouar Z.R., Ratts T.E., Cunningham B.R., et al.: Altered ventricular diastolic properties in borderline hypertension: Effect of sodium intake. *Circulation* 64(IV):322, 1981.
56. Sullivan J.M., Prewitt R.L., Josephs J.A.: Attenuation of the microcirculation in young patients with high output labile hypertension. *Hypertension* 5:844–851, 1983.
57. Meerson F.: The myocardium in hyperfunction, hypertrophy, and failure. *Circ. Res.* 25(Suppl. 2):1–54, 1969.
58. Ledingham J.M., Cohen R.D.: The role of the heart in the pathogenesis of renal hypertension. *Lancet* 2:979–981, 1963.
59. Guyton A.C., Granger H.J., Coleman T.G.: Autoregulation of the total systemic circulation and its relation to control of cardiac output and arterial pressure. *Circ. Res.* 28(Suppl. 1):93–97, 1971.
60. Tarazi R.C.: Hemodynamic role of extracellular fluid in hypertension. *Circ. Res.* 38(Suppl. II):II-73–II-83, 1976.
61. Sullivan J.M., Schoeneberger A.A., Ratts T.E., et al.: Short-term therapy of severe hypertension. Hemodynamic correlates of the antihypertensive response in man. *Arch. Intern. Med.* 139:1233–1239, 1979.
62. Ambard L., Beaujard E.: Cause de l'hypertension arterielle. *Arch. Gen. Med.* 1:520–533, 1904.

63. Sasaki N.: The relationship of salt intake to hypertension in the Japanese. *Geriatrics* 19:735–744, 1964.
64. Kempner W.: Treatment of kidney disease and hypertensive vascular disease with rice diet. *N.C. Med. J.* 5:125–133, 1944.
65. Murphy R.J.F.: The effect of "rice diet" on plasma volume and extracellular fluid space in hypertensive subjects. *J. Clin. Invest.* 29:912–917, 1950.
66. Parijs J., Joosens J.V., Vander Linden L., et al.: Moderate sodium restriction and diuretics in the treatment of hypertension. *Am. Heart J.* 85:22–34, 1973.
67. Luft F.C., Weinberger M.H., Grim C.E., et al.: Sodium sensitivity in normotensive human subjects. *Ann. Intern. Med.* 98:758–762, 1983.
68. Coleman T.G., Buyton A.C.: Hypertension caused by salt loading in the dog. III. Onset transients of cardiac output and other variables. *Circ. Res.* 25:153–160, 1969.
69. Dahl L.K.: Salt and hypertension. *Am. J. Clin. Nutr.* 25:231–244, 1972.
70. Bianchi G., DiFrancesco G.F., et al.: Blood pressure changes produced by kidney cross-transplantation between spontaneously hypertensive rats (SHR) and normotensive rats (NR). *Clin. Sci.* 47:435–448, 1974.
71. Dahl L.K., Heine M., Thompson K.: Genetic influence of the kidneys on blood pressure. Evidence from chronic renal homografts in rats with opposite predispositions to hypertension. *Circ. Res.* 34:94–101, 1974.
72. Dahl L.K., Knudsen K.D., Iwai J.: Humeral transmission of hypertension: evidence from parabiosis. *Circ. Res.* 24 & 25(Suppl.)I-21–I-33, 1969.
73. Tobian L., Ishii M., Duke M.: Relationship of cytoplasmic granules in renal papillary interstitial cells to "post-salt" hypertension. *J. Lab. Clin. Med.* 73:309–319, 1969.
74. Ganguli M., Tobian L., Iwai J.: Cardiac output and peripheral resistance in strains of rats sensitive and resistant to NaCl hypertension. *Hypertension* 1:3–7, 1979.
75. Kisch B.: Electron microscopy of the atrium of the heart. *Exp. Med. Surg.* 14:99–112, 1956.
76. deBold A.J.: Heart atria granularity effects changes in water-electrolyte balance. *Proc. Soc. Exp. Biol. Med.* 161:508–511, 1979.
77. deBold A.J., Borenstein H.B., Veress A.T., et al.: A rapid and potent natriuretic response to intravenous injection of atrial myocardial extract in rats. *Life Sci.* 28:89–94, 1981.
78. Sonnenburg H., Cupples W.A., deBold A.J., et al.: Intrarenal localization of the natriuretic effect of cardiac atrial extract. *Can. J. Physiol. Pharmacol.* 60:1149–1152, 1982.
79. Mark A.L.: The Bezold-Jarisch reflex revisited: Clinical implications of inhibitory reflexes originating in the heart. *J. Am. Coll. Cardiol.* 1:90–102, 1983.
80. De Wardener H.E., Clarkson E.M.: The natriuretic hormone: Recent developments. *Clin. Sci.* 63:415–420, 1982.
81. Blaustein M.P.: Sodium ions, calcium ions, blood pressure regulation, and hypertension: A reassessment and a hypothesis. *Am. J. Physiol.* 232:C165–C173, 1977.
82. Hamlyn J.M., Ringel R., Schaeffer J., et al.: A circulating inhibitor of (Na + K) ATPase associated with essential hypertension. *Nature* 300:650–652, 1982.

83. Kirkendall W.M., Connor W.E., Abboud F., et al.: The effect of dietary sodium on the blood pressure of normal man, in Genest J., Koiw E. (eds.): *Hypertension '72*. Berlin, Springer-Verlag, 1972, pp. 360–374.

84. Mark A.L., Lawton W.J., Abboud F.M., et al.: Effects of high and low sodium intake on arterial pressure and forearm vascular resistance in borderline hypertension. *Circ. Res.* 36(Suppl. 1):I-194–I-198, 1975.

85. Frohlich E.D., Tarazi R.C., Dustan H.P.: Reexamination of the hemodynamics of hypertension. *Am. J. Med. Sci.* 257:9–23, 1969.

86. Julius S., Pascual A.V., Reilly K., et al.: Abnormalities of plasma volume in borderline hypertension. *Arch. Intern. Med.* 127:116–119, 1971.

87. Sullivan J.M., Ratts T.E., Schoeneberger A.A., et al.: The effect of diet on echocardiographic left ventricular dimensions in normal man. *Am. J. Clin. Nutr.* 32:2410–2415, 1979.

88. Sullivan J.M., Ratts T.E., Taylor J.C., et al.: Hemodynamic effects of dietary sodium in man. A preliminary report. *Hypertension* 2:506–514, 1980.

89. Sullivan J.M., Ratts T.E.: Hemodynamic mechanism of adaptation to chronic high sodium intake in normal man. *Hypertension* 5:814, 1983.

90. Onesti G., Kim K., Greco J., et al.: Blood pressure regulation in end-stage renal disease and anephric man. *Circ. Res.* 36(Suppl. 1):I-145–I-152, 1975.

91. Bravo E., Tarazi R., Dustan H.: Multifactorial analysis of chronic hypertension induced by electrolyte-active steroids in trained unanesthetized dogs. *Circ. Res.* 40 (Suppl. 1):I-140–I-145, 1977.

92. Berecek K., Bohr D.: Whole body vascular reactivity during the development of deoxycorticosterone acetate hypertension in the pig. *Circ. Res.* 42:764–771, 1978.

93. Luft F.C., Weinberger W.H., Grim C.E.: Sodium sensitivity and resistance in normotensive humans. *Am. J. Med.* 72:726–736, 1982.

94. Langford H.G.: Dietary potassium and epidemiologic data. *Ann. Intern. Med.* 98:770–772, 1983.

95. Emanuel D.A., Scott J.B., Haddy F.J.: Effect of potassium on small and large blood vessels of the dog forelimb. *Am. J. Physiol.* 197:637–642, 1959.

96. Lowe R.D., Thompson J.W.: The effect of intra-arterial potassium chloride infusion upon forearm blood flow in man. *J. Physiol.* (Lond.) 162:69P–70P, 1962.

97. Overbeck H.W., Derifield R.S., Pamnani M.B.: Attenuated vasodilator responses to K in essential hypertensive men. *J. Clin. Invest.* 53(3):678–686, 1974.

98. Luft F.C., Rankin L.I., Bloch R., et al.: Cardiovascular and humoral responses to extremes of sodium intake in normal black and white men. *Circulation* 60(3):697–706, 1979.

99. MacGregor G.A., Smith S.J., Marhandu N.D., et al.: Moderate potassium supplementation in essential hypertension. *Lancet* 2:567–570, 1982.

100. Gibson D.G., Trail T.A., Hall R.J.C., et al.: Echocardiographic features of secondary left ventricular hypertrophy. *Br. Heart J.* 41:54–59, 1979.

101. Ratts T.E., Addington B., Gerlach P., et al.: Echocardiographic-clinical correlation of heart failure in hypertension. *J. Am. Coll. Cardiol.* 3:592, 1984.

102. Engelman K., Portnoy B., Sjoersdma A.: Plasma catecholamine concentration in patients with hypertension. *Circ. Res.* 27:I-141–I-146, 1970.

103. DeQuatro V., Chan S.: Raised plasma-catecholamines in some patients with primary hypertension. *Lancet* 1:806–809, 1972.
104. Louis W.J., Doyle A.E., Anavekar S.: Plasma norepinephrine levels in essential hypertension. *N. Engl. J. Med.* 288:599–601, 1973.
105. Stone R.A., Gunnells J.C., Robinson R.R., et al.: Dopamine-beta-hydroxylase in primary and secondary hypertension. *Circ. Res.* 34:I-47–I-56, 1974.
106. Louis W.J., Doyle A.E., Anavekar S.N., et al.: Plasma catecholamine, dopamine-beta-hydroxylase and renin levels in essential hypertension. *Circ. Res.* 34:1–57, 1974.
107. Engelman K., Portnoy B., Lovenberg W.: A sensitive and specific double isotope derivative method for the determination of catecholamine in biological specimens. *Am. J. Med. Sci.* 255:259–268, 1968.
108. DeQuattro V., Miura J.; Neurogenic factors in human hypertension: Mechanism or myth? in Laragh J.H. (ed.): *Hypertension Manual.* New York, Yorke Medical Books, 1972, pp. 277–312.
109. Gitlow S.E., Mendlowitz M., Wilk E.K., et al.: Plasma clearance of d_1-beta-H_3-norepinephrine in normal human subjects and patients with essential hypertension. *J. Clin. Invest.* 43:2009–2015, 1964.
110. DeQuattro V., Sjoerdsma A.: Catecholamine turnovers in normotensive and hypertensive man: Effects of antiadrenegic drug. *J. Clin. Invest.* 47:2359–2373, 1968.
111. Tigerstedt R., Bergman P.G.: Niere and Dreishauf. *Skand. Arch. Physiol.* 8:223–271, 1898.
112. Goldblatt H., Lynch J., Hanzal R.F., et al.: Studies on experimental hypertension. I. The production of persistent elevation of systolic blood pressure by means of renal ischemia. *J. Exp. Med.* 59:347–379, 1934.
113. Page, I.H.: On the nature of the pressor action of renin. *J. Exp. Med.* 70:521–542, 1939.
114. Braun-Menendez E., Fasciolo J.C., Leloir L.F., et al.: La substancia hypertensova de la sangre del finon isquemiado. *Revta Soc. Argent. Biol.* 15:420–435, 1939.
115. Simpson S.A., Tait J.F., Wettstein A., et al.: Isolierung eines neuen kristallisierten hormons aus nebennieren mit besonders hoher wieksamkeit aus den meneral-stofswechsel. *Experientia* (Basel) 9:333–335, 1953.
116. Laragh J.H., Ungers M., Kelly W.G., et al.: Hypotensive agents and pressor substances. The effect of epinephrine, norepinephrine, angiotensin II and others on the secretory rate of aldosterone in man. *J.A.M.A.* 174:234–240, 1960.
117. Genest J., Nowaczynski W., Koiw E., et al.: Adrenocorticoid function in essential hypertension, in Boch K.D., Cottier P.T. (eds.): *Essential Hypertension,* Berlin, Springer-Verlag, 1960, pp. 126–146.
118. Blair-West J.R., Coghlan J.P., Denton D.A., et al.: The effect of heptapeptide (2-8) and hexapeptide (3-8) fragments of angiotensin II on aldosterone secretion. *J. Clin. Endocrinol. Metab.* 32:575–578, 1971.
119. Davis J.O.: What signals the kidney to release renin? *Circ. Res.* 28:301–306, 1971.
120. Tobian L., Tomboulian A., Janecek J.: Effect of high perfusion pressures on the granulation of juxtaglomerular cells in an isolated kidney. *J. Clin. Invest.* 38:605–610, 1959.

121. Vander A.J.: Effect of catecholamines and the renal nerves on renin secretion in anesthetized dogs. *Am. J. Physiol.* 209:659–662, 1965.
122. Skinner S.L., McCubbin J.W., Page, I.H.: Control of renin secretion. *Circ. Res.* 15:64–76, 1964.
123. Vander A.J., Miller, R.: Control of renin secretion in the anesthetized dog. *Am. J. Physiol.* 207:537–546, 1964.
124. Brown J.J., Davies D.L., Lever A.R., et al.: Plasma renin concentration in human hypertension. I. Relationship between renin, sodium, and potassium. *Br. Med. J.* 3:144–148, 1965.
125. Veyrat R., Brunner J.R., Manning E.L., et al.: Inhibition de l'activité de la reniné plasmatique par le potassium. *J. Urol. Nephrol.* (Paris)73:271–275, 1967.
126. Vander A.J., Greelhoed G.W.: Inhibition of renin secretion by angiotensin II. *Proc. Soc. Exp. Biol. Med.* 120:399–403, 1965.
127. Wathen R.L., Kingsbury W.S., Stouder D.A., et al.: Effects of infusion of catecholamines and angiotensin II on renin release in anethetized dogs. *Amer. J. Physiol.* 209:1012–1024, 1965.
128. Helmer O.M., Griffith R.S.: The effect of the administration of estrogens on the renin-substrate (hypertensinogen) content of rat plasma. *Endocrinology* 51:421–426, 1952.
129. Robb C.A., Davis J.O., Johnson C.E., et al.: Effect of deoxycorticosterone on plasma renin activity in conscious dogs. *Am. J. Physiol.* 216:884–889, 1969.
130. Vander A.J.: Inhibition of renin release in the dog by vasopressin and vasotocin. *Circ. Res.* 23:605–609, 1968.
131. Larsson C., Weber P., Änggard E.: Arachidonic acid increases and indomethacine decreases plasma renin activity in the rabbit. *Eur. J. Pharmacol.* 28:391–394, 1974.
132. Henrich W.L.: Role of the prostaglandins in renin secretion. *Kidney Int.* 19:822–830, 1981.
133. Gotshall R.W., Davis J.O., Shade R.E., et al.: Effects of renal denervation on renin release in sodium depleted dogs. *Am. J. Physiol.* 225 (No. 2):344–349, 1973.
134. Assaykeen T.A., Clayton P.L., Goldfien A., et al.: Effect of alpha and beta-adrenergic blocking agents on the renin response to hypoglycemia and epinephrine in dogs. *Endocrinology* 87:1318–1322, 1970.
135. Passo S.S., Assaykeen T.A., Goldfien A., et al.: Effect of alpha and beta adrenergic blocking agents on the increase in renin secretion produced by stimulation of the medulla oblongata. *Neuroendocrinology* 7:97–104, (1971a).
136. Winer N., Walkerkorst W.G.: Effect of cyclic AMP, sympathomimetic amines and adrenergic antagonists on renin secretion. *Circ. Res.* 29:239–248, 1971.
137. Winer N.: Mechanism of increased renin secretion associated with adrenalectomy, hemorrhage, renal artery constriction and sodium depletion, in Genest J., Koiw E. (eds.): *Hypertension '72*. Berlin, Heidelberg, New York, Springer-Verlag New York, 1972, pp. 25–36.
138. Tanigawa H., Allison D.J., Assaykeen T.A.: A comparison of the effects of various catecholamines on plasma renin activity alone and in the pres-

ence of adrenergic blocking agents, in Genest J., Koiw E. (eds.): *Hypertension '72*. Berlin, Heidelberg, New York, Springer-Verlag New York, 1972, pp. 37–44.

139. Ganong W.F.: Effect of sympathetic activity and ACTH on renin and aldosterone secretion, in Genest J., Koiw E. (eds.): *Hypertension '72*. Berlin, Heidelberg, New York, Springer-Verlag New York, 1972, pp. 4–13.

140. Sullivan J.M., Adams D.F., Hollenberg N.K.: Beta-blockade in essential hypertension. Reduced renin release despite renal vasoconstriction. *Circ. Res.* 39:532–536, 1976.

141. Buhler F.R., Laragh J.H., Baer L., et al.: Propranolol inhibition of renin secretion. *N. Engl. J. Med.* 287:1209–1214, 1972.

142. Michelakis A.M., McAllister R.G.: The effect of chronic adrenergic receptor blockade on plasma renin activity in man. *J. Clin. Endocrinol. Metab.* 34:386–394, 1972.

143. Winer N., Chokski D.S., Yoon M.S., et al.: Adrenergic receptor mediation of renin secretion. *J. Clin. Endocrinol. Metab.* 29:1168–1175, 1969.

144. Bravo E.L., Tarazi R.C., Dustan H.P.: Beta-adrenergic blockade in diuretic-treated patients with essential hypertension. *N. Engl. J. Med.* 292:66–70, 1975.

145. Bravo E.L., Tarazi R.C., Dustan H.P.: On the mechanism of suppressed plasma renin activity during beta-adrenergic blockade with propranolol. *J. Lab. Clin. Med.* 83:119–128, 1974.

146. Couch N.P., Sullivan J.M., Crane C.: The predictive accuracy of renal vein renin activity in the surgery of renovascular hypertension. *Surgery* 79:70–76, 1976.

147. Brunner H.R., Laragh J.H., Baer L., et al.: Essential hypertension: Renin and aldosterone, heart attack and stroke. *N. Engl. J. Med.* 286:441–449, 1972.

148. Channick B.J., Adlin E.V., Marks A.D.: Suppressed plasma renin activity in hypertension. *Arch. Intern. Med.* 123:131–140, 1969.

149. Drayer J.I.M., Kloppenborg P.W.C., Benraad T.J.: Detection of low-renin hypertension: Evaluation of outpatient renin-stimulating methods, *Clin. Sci.* 48:(2)91–96, 1975.

150. Dunn M.J., Tannen R.L.: Low-renin hypertension. *Kidney Int.* 5:317–325, 1974.

151. Laragh J.H.: Vasoconstriction-volume analysis for understanding and treating hypertension: The use of renin and aldosterone profiles. *Am. J. Med.* 55:261–274, 1973.

152. Woods, J.W., Liddle G.W., Stant E.G. Jr., et al.: Effect of an adrenal inhibitor in hypertensive patients with suppressed renin. *Arch. Intern. Med.* 123:366–370, 1969.

153. Carey R.M., Douglas J.G., Schjweikert J.R., et al.: The syndrome of essential hypertension and suppressed plasma renin activity: Normalization of blood pressure with spironolactone. *Arch. Intern. Med.* 130:849–854, 1972.

154. Woods J.W., Pittman A.W., et al.: Renin profiling in hypertension and its use in treatment with propranolol and chlorthalidone. *N. Engl. J. Med.* 294:1137–1143, 1976.

155. Weidman P., Hirsch D., Maxwell M.H., et al.: Plasma renin and blood

pressure during treatment with methyldopa. *Am. J. Cardiol.* 34:671–676, 1974.

156. Green L.J., Camargo A.C.M., Krieger E.M., et al.: Inhibition of the conversion of angiotensin I to II and potentiation of bradykinin by small peptides present in Bothrops jararaca venom. *Circ. Res.* 31(suppl. 2):62–71, 1972.

157. Ondetti M.A., Rubin R., Cushman D.W.: Design of specific inhibitors of angiotensin-converting enzyme: New class of orally active antihypertensive agents. *Science* 196:441–444, 1977.

158. Sweet C.S., Gross D.M., Arbegast P.T., et al.: Antihypertensive activity of N-[(S)-1-(Ethoxycarbonyl)-3-phenylpropyl]-L-ala-L-pro (MK-42), an orally active converting enzyme inhibitor. *J. Pharmacol. Exp. Ther.* 216:63–69, 1981.

159. Ulm E.H., Hichens M., Gomez H.J., et al.: Enalapril maleate and a lysine analogue (MK-521) disposition in man. *Br. J. Clin. Pharmacol.* 14:357–362, 1982.

160. Pals D.T., Mascucci F.D., Sipos F., et al.: A specific competitive antagonist of the vascular action of angiotensin II. *Circ. Res.* 29:664–672, 1971.

161. Brunner H.R., Gavras H.: Clinical implications of renin in the hypertensive patient. *J.A.M.A.* 233:1091–1093, 1975.

162. Streeten D.H.P., Anderson G.H., Dalakos T.G.: Angiotensin blockade: Its clinical significance. *Am. J. Med.* 60:817–824, 1976.

163. Hedqvist P.: Studies on the effect of prostaglandins E_1 and E_2 on the sympathetic neuromuscular transmission in some animal tissues. *Acta Physiol. Scand. (Suppl.)* 345:1–40, 1970.

164. DuCharme D.W., Weeks J.R., Montgomery R.C.: Studies on the mechanism of the hypertensive effect of prostaglandin F_2 alpha. *J. Pharmacol. Exp. Ther.* 160:1–10, 1968.

165. Malik K.U., McGiff J.C.: Cardiovascular actions of prostaglandins, in Karim S.M.M. (ed.): *Prostaglandins: Physiological, Pharmacological and Pathological Aspects.* Lancaster, England, MTP Press Ltd., 1976, pp. 103–200.

166. Nakano J.M., McCurdy J.R.: Cardiovascular effects of prostaglandin E_1. *J. Pharmacol. Exp. Ther.* 156:538–586, 1967.

167. Siren A.L.: Differences in the central actions of arachidonic acid and prostaglandin F_2 alpha between spontaneously hypertensive and normotensive rats. *Life Sci.* 30(6):503–513, 1982.

168. Terragno D.A., Crowshaw K., Terragno N.A., et al.: Prostaglandin synthesis by bovine mesenteric arteries and veins. *Circ. Res.* 36–37(Suppl.I):I-76–I-80, 1975.

169. Terragno N.A., Terragno D.A., McGiff J.C.: Contribution of prostaglandins to the renal circulation in conscious, anesthetized and laparotomized dogs. *Circ. Res.* 40:590–595, 1977.

170. Grantham J.J., Orloff J.: Effect of prostaglandin E_1 on the permeability response of the isolated collecting tubule to vasopressin, adenosine 3′, 5′-monophosphate, and theophylline. *J. Clin. Invest.* 47:1154–1161, 1968.

171. Gryglewski R.J., Korbut R., Ocetkiewicz A.: Generation of prostacyclin by lungs in vivo and its release into the arterial circulation. *Nature* 273:765–767, 1978.

172. Moncada S., Korbut R., Bunting S., et al.: Prostacyclin is a circulating hormone. *Nature* 273:767–768, 1978.

173. Armstrong J.M., Lattimer N., Moncada S., et al.: Comparison of the vasodepressor effects of prostacyclin and 6-oxo-prostaglandin F_1-alpha with those of prostaglandin E_2 in rats and rabbits. *Br. J. Pharmacol.* 62:125–130, 1978.

174. Dusting G.J., Moncada S., Vane J.R.: Recirculation of prostacyclin (PGI$_2$) in the dog. *Br. J. Pharmacol.* 64:315–320, 1978.

175. McGiff J.C., Terragno N.A., Strand J.C., et al.: Selective passage of prostaglandins across the lung. *Nature* 223:742–745, 1969.

176. Carr A.A.: Hemodynamic and renal effects of a prostaglandin, PGA$_1$ in subjects with essential hypertension. *Am. J. Med. Sci.* 259:21–26, 1970.

177. Zusman R.M., Caldwell B.V., Mulrow P.J., et al.: The role of prostaglandin A in the control of sodium homeostasis and blood pressure. *Prostaglandins* 3:679–690, 1973.

178. Frolich J.C., Sweetman B.J., Carr K., et al.: Assessment of the levels of PGA$_2$ in human plasma by gas chromatography-mass spectrometry. *Prostaglandins* 10:185–195, 1975.

179. Granstrom E.: Metabolism of prostaglandins, in Berti F., Samuelsson B., Velo G.P. (eds.): *Prostaglandins and Thromboxanes*. New York, Plenum Press, 1977, pp. 75–83.

180. Piper P.J., Vane J.R.: Release of additional factors in anaphylaxis and its antagonism by anti-inflammatory drugs. *Nature* 223:29–35, 1969.

181. Hamberg M., Samuelsson B.: Prostaglandin endoperoxides. Novel transformations of arachidonic acid in human platelets. *Proc. Natl. Acad. Sci. USA* 71:3400–3404, 1974.

182. Hamberg M., Svensson J., Samuelsson B.: Thromboxanes: a new group of biologically active compounds derived from prostaglandin endoperoxides. *Proc. Natl. Acad. Sci. USA* 72:2994–2998, 1975.

183. Bunting S., Gryglewski R., Moncada S., et al.: Arterial walls generate from prostaglandin endoperoxides a substance (prostaglandin X) which relaxes strips of mesenteric and coeliac arteries and inhibits platelet aggregation. *Prostaglandins* 12:897–913, 1976.

184. Moncada S., Higgs E.A., Vane J.R.: Human arterial and venous tissues generate prostacyclin (prostaglandin X), a potent inhibitor of platelet aggregation. *Lancet* 1:18–20, 1977.

185. Aiken J.W.: Effects of prostaglandin synthesis inhibitors on angiotensin tachyphylaxis in the isolated coeliac and mesenteric arteries of the rabbit. *Pol. J. Pharmacol. Pharm.* 26:217–227, 1974.

186. Mullane K.M., Moncada S.: Prostacyclin release and the modulation of some vasoactive hormones. *Prostaglandins* 20:25–49, 1980.

187. Grodzinska L., Gruglewski R.J.: Angiotensin-induced release of prostacyclin from perfused organs. *Pharmacol. Res. Commun.* 12:339–347, 1980.

188. Needleman P., Bronson S.D., Wyche A., et al.: Cardiac and renal prostaglandin I$_2$. Biosynthesis and biologic effects in isolated perfused rabbit tissue. *J. Clin. Invest.* 61:839–849, 1978.

189. Malik K.U.: Prostaglandin-mediated inhibition of the vasoconstrictor responses of the isolated perfused rat splenic vasculature to adrenergic stimuli. *Circ. Res.* 43(2):225–233, 1978.

190. Nasjletti A., Malik K.U.: Interrelations between prostaglandins and vasoconstrictor hormones: Contribution to blood pressure regulation. *Med. Clin. No. Am.* 65:881–889, 1981.

191. Beilin L.J., Bhattacharya J.: The effect of prostaglandin synthesis inhibitors on renal blood flow distribution in conscious rabbits. *J. Physiol.* 269:395–405, 1977.
192. Colina-Chourio J., McGiff J.C., Nasjletti A.: Effect of indomethacin on blood pressure in the normotensive unanesthetized rabbit: Possible relation to prostaglandin synthesis inhibition. *Clin. Sci.* 57:359–365, 1979.
193. Muirhead E.E., Brooks B., Brosius W.L.: Indomethacin and blood pressure control. *J. Lab. Clin. Med.* 88:578–583, 1976.
194. Romero J.C., Strong J.C.: The effect of indomethacin blockade of prostaglandin synthesis on blood pressure of normal rabbits and rabbits with renovascular hypertension. *Circ. Res.* 40:35–41, 1977.
195. Chrysant S.G., Townsend S.M., Morgan P.R.: The effects of salt and meclofenamate administration on the hypertension of spontaneously hypertensive rats. *Clin. Exp. Hypertens.* 1:381–391, 1978.
196. Pugsley D.J., Bullins R., Beilin L.J.: Renal prostaglandin synthesis in hypertension induced by deoxycorticosterone and sodium chloride in the rat. *Clin. Sci.* 51 (Suppl 3):253s–256s, 1976.
197. McQueen D., Bell K.: The effects of prostaglandin E_1 and sodium meclofenamate on blood pressure in renal hypertensive rats. *Eur. J. Pharmacol.* 37:223–235, 1976.
198. Yun J., Kelly G., Bartter F.C.: Effect of indomethacin on renal function and plasma renin activity in dogs with chronic renovascular hypertension. *Nephron* 24:278–282, 1979.
199. Wennmalm A.: Hypertensive effect of the prostaglandin synthesis inhibitor indomethacin. *IRCS (Research on: Endocrine System)* 2:1099, 1974.
200. Nowak J., Wennmalm A.: Influence of indomethacin and prostaglandin E_1 on total and regional blood flow in man. *Acta Physiol. Scand.* 102:484–491, 1978.
201. Negus P., Tannen R.L., Dunn M.J.: Indomethacin potentiates the vasoconstrictor actions of angiotensin II in normal man. *Prostaglandins* 12:175–180, 1976.
202. Patak R.B., Mookerjee C., Bentzel P., et al.: Antagonism of the effects of furosemide by indomethacin in normal and hypertensive man. *Prostaglandins* 10:649–659, 1975.
203. Durão V., Prata M.M., Goncalves L.M.P.: Modification of antihypertensive effect of beta-adrenoceptor-blocking agents by inhibition of endogenous prostaglandin synthesis. *Lancet* 2:1005–1007, 1977.
204. De Jong P.E., Donker A.J.M., Vand der Wall E., et al.: Effect of indomethacin in two siblings with a renin-dependent hypertension, hyperaldosteronism and hypokalemia. *Nephron* 25:47–52, 1980.
205. Rioux F., Quirion R., Regoli D.: The role of prostaglandins in hypertension. I. The release of prostaglandins by aortic strips of renal, DOCA-salt, and spontaneously hypertensive rats. *Can. J. Physiol. Pharmacol.* 55:1330–1338, 1977.
206. Limas C.J., Limas C.: Prostaglandin metabolism in the kidneys of spontaneously hypertensive rats. *Am. J. Physiol.* 233(1):H87–H92, 1977.
207. Pace-Asciak C.R., Carrara M.C., Rangaraj G., et al.: Enhanced formation of PGI_2, a potent hypotensive substance, by aortic rings and homogenates of the spontaneously hypertensive rat. *Prostaglandins* 15(6):1005–1012, 1978.

208. Pipili E., Poyser N.L.: Release of prostaglandins I_2 and E_2 from the perfused mesenteric arterial bed of normotensive and hypertensive rats. Effects of sympathetic nerve stimulation and norepinephrine administration. *Prostaglandins* 23(4):543–549, 1982.

209. McGiff J.C., Crowshaw K., Terragno N.A.: Renal prostaglandins: possible regulators of the renal actions of pressure hormones. *Nature* 227:1255–1257, 1970.

210. Aiken J.W., Vane J.R.: Intrarenal prostaglandin release attenuates the renal vasoconstrictor activity of angiotensin. *J. Pharmacol. Exp. Ther.* 183:678–687, 1973.

211. Lonigro A.J., Itskovitz H.D., Crowshaw K., et al.: Dependency of renal blood flow on prostaglandin synthesis in the dog. *Circ. Res.* 32:712–717, 1973.

212. Beaty O. III, Donald D.E.: Contribution of prostaglandins to muscle blood flow in anesthetized dogs at rest, during exercise, and following inflow occlusion. *Circ. Res.* 44:67–75, 1979.

213. Ishii M., Mehara Y., Hirata Y., Atarashi K., et al.: Effects of norepinephrine infusion on systemic hemodynamics and plasma 6-keto-prostaglandin F1-alpha in normotensive subjects and patients with essential hypertension. *Jpn. Circ. J.* 46(5):494–502, 1982.

214. Chaignon M., Ruffie M.L., Lucsko M., et al.: Prostacyclin infusion in hypertension: Acute hemodynamic and hormonal effects. *N. Engl. J. Med.* 307:559, 1982.

215. Lima D.R., Turner P.: Beta-blocking drugs increase responsiveness to prostacyclin in hypertensive patients. *Lancet* 2:444, 1982.

216. Malmsten C., Hamberg M., Svensson J., et al.: Physiological role of an endoperoxide in human platelets: hemostatic defect due to platelet cyclo-oxygenase deficiency. *Proc. Natl. Acad. Sci. USA* 72:1446–1450, 1975.

217. Wong P.Y-K., Sun F.F., McGiff J.C.: Metabolism of prostacyclin in blood vessels. *J. Biol. Chem.* 253:5555–5557, 1978.

218. Hensby C.N., Dollery C.T., Barnes P.J., et al.: Production of 6-oxo-PGF_1-alpha by human lung in vivo. *Lancet* 2:1162–1163, 1979.

219. Szczeklik A., Gryglewski R.J., Nizankowska E., et al.: Pulmonary and anti-platelet effects of intravenous and inhaled prostacyclin in man. *Prostaglandins* 16:651–659, 1978.

220. Gimeno M.F., Sterin-Borda L., Borda E.S., et al.: Human plasma transforms prostacyclin (PGI_2) into a platelet antiaggregatory substance which contracts isolated bovine coronary arteries. *Prostaglandins* 19:907–916, 1980.

221. Hoult J.R.S., Lofts F.J., Moore P.K.: Stability of prostacyclin in plasma and its transformation by platelets to a stable spasmogenic product. *Proceedings Br. J. Pharmacol. Soc.* 68 (abstract), 1981.

222. Wong P.Y-K., Lee W.H., Chao P.H-W., et al.: Metabolism of prostacyclin by 0-hydroxyprostaglandin dehydrogenase in human platelets. *J. Biol. Chem.* 255:9021–9024, 1980.

223. Hollenberg N.K., Solomon H.S., Adams D.F., et al.: Renal vascular responses to angiotensin and norepinephrine in normal man. *Circ. Res.* 31:750–757, 1972.

224. Meneely G.R., Ball C.O.T., Youmans J.B.: Chronic sodium chloride tox-

icity: the protective effect of added potassium chloride. *Ann. Intern. Med.* 47:263–273, 1957.

225. Itskovitz H.D., McGiff J.C.: Hormonal regulation of the renal circulation. *Circ. Res.* 34 (Suppl. I):I-65–I-73, 1974.

226. Vane J.R.: The release and fate of vasoactive hormones in the circulation. *Br. J. Pharmacol.* 35:209–242, 1969.

227. Muirhead E.E., Leach B.C., Byers L.W., et al.: Antihypertensive neutral renomedullary lipids (ANRD), in Fisher J.W. (ed.): *Kidney Hormones.* New York, Academic Press, 1971, pp. 485–506.

228. McGiff J.C., Crowshaw K., Terragno N.A., et al.: Renal prostaglandins: possible regulators in the renal actions of pressor hormones. *Nature* 227:1255–1257, 1970.

229. Dunn M.J.: Renal prostaglandin synthesis in the spontaneously hypertensive rat. *J. Clin. Invest.* 58:862–870, 1976.

230. Pace-Asciak C.P.: Decreased renal prostaglandin catabolism precedes onset of hypertension in the developing spontaneously hypertensive rat. *Nature* 263:510–512, 1976.

231. Stygles V.G., Reinke D.A., Rickert D.E., et al.: Increased blood pressure in the SHR is not related to a deficit in renomedullary PGE_2. *Experientia* 15:1025–1026, 1978.

232. Ahnfelt-Rønne I., Arrigoni-Martelli E.: Increased PGF_2-alpha synthesis in renal papilla of spontaneously hypertensive rats. *Biochem. Pharmacol.* 27:2363–2367, 1978.

233. Armstrong J.M., Blackwell G.J., Flower R.J., et al.: Genetic hypertension in rats is accompanied by a defect in renal prostaglandin catabolism. *Nature* (London) 260:582–586, 1976.

234. Tan S.Y., Sweet P., Mulrow P.J.: Impaired renal production of prostaglandin E_2: a newly identified lesion in human essential hypertension. *Prostaglandins* 15(1):139–150, 1978.

235. Clive D.M., Stoff J.S.: Renal syndromes associated with nonsteroidal anti-inflammatory drugs. *New Engl. J. Med.* 310:563–572, 1984.

236. McGiff J.C., Crowshaw K., Terragno N.A., et al.: Release of a prostaglandin-like substance into renal venous blood in response to angiotensin II. *Circ. Res.* 26–27(Suppl I):I-121–I-130, 1970.

237. Itskovitz H.D., Terragno N.A., McGiff J.C.: Effect of a renal prostaglandin on distribution of blood flow in the isolated canine kidney. *Circ. Res.* 34:770–776, 1974.

238. Larsson C., Änggard E.: Regional differences in the formation and metabolism of prostaglandins in the rabbit kidney. *Eur. J. Pharmacol.* 21:30–36, 1973.

239. Terragno N.A., McGiff J.C., Terragno A.: Synthesis of prostaglandin by vascular and nonvascular renal tissues and the presence of an endogenous prostaglandin synthesis inhibitor in the cortex, in Vargastig B.B. (ed.): *Advances in Pharmacology and Therapeutics, vol. 4, Prostaglandins and Immunopharmacology.* Oxford, Pergamon Press, 1978, pp. 39–46.

240. Janszen F.H.A., Nugteren D.H.: Histochemical localisation of prostaglandin synthetase. *Histochemie* 27:159–164, 1971.

241. Berl T., Raz A., Wald H., et al.: Prostaglandin synthesis inhibition and the action of vasopressin: Studies in man and rat. *Am. J. Physiol.* 232(6):F529–F537, 1977.

242. Tobian L., Ganguli M., Johnson M.A., et al.: Influence of renal prostaglandins and dietary lineoleate on hypertension in Dahl S rats. *Hypertension* 4:325–328, 1982.
243. Frölich J.C., Hollifield J.W., Dormois J.C., et al.: Suppression of plasma renin activity by indomethacin in man. *Clin. Res.* 39:447–452, 1976.
244. Weber P.C., Larsson C., Anggard E., et al.: Stimulation of renin release from rabbit renal cortex by arachidonic acid and prostaglandin endoperoxides. *Circ. Res.* 39:868–874, 1976.
245. Whorton A.R., Misono K., Hollifield J., et al.: Prostaglandins and renin release: Stimulation of renin release from rabbit renal cortical slices by PGI$_2$. *Prostaglandins* 14:1095–1104, 1977.
246. Hoult J.R., Moore P.K.: Pathways of prostaglandin F$_2$-alpha metabolism in mammalian kidneys. *Br. J. Pharmacol.* 61:615–616, 1977.
247. Spokas E.G., Ferreri N.R., Wong P.Y-K., et al.: Effect of 6-keto prostaglandin E$_1$ (6-keto-PGE$_1$) on renin release from rabbit renal cortical slices. *Circulation* 62:III–287(Abstract).
248. Jackson E.K., Herzer W.A., Zimmerman J.B., et al.: 6-keto prostaglandin E$_1$ is more potent than prostaglandin I$_2$ as a renal vasodilator and renin secretagogue. *J. Pharmacol. Exper. Ther.* 216:24–27, 1981.
249. Bartter F.C., Pronove P., Gill J.R. Jr., et al.: Hyperplasia of the juxtaglomerular complex with hyperaldosteronism and hypokalemic alkalosis. A new syndrome. *Am. J. Med.* 33:811–828, 1962.
250. Gill J.R., Frölich J.C., Bowden R.E., et al.: Bartter's syndrome: a disorder characterized by high urinary prostaglandins and a dependence of hyperreninemia on prostaglandin synthesis. *Am. J. Med.* 61:43–51, 1976.
251. Halushka P.V., Wohltmann H., Privitera P.J.: Bartter's syndrome: urinary prostaglandin E-like material and kallikrein; indomethacin effects. *Ann. Intern. Med.* 87:281–286, 1977.
252. Verberckmoes R., van Damme B., Clement J., et al.: Bartter's syndrome with hyperplasia of renomedullary cells: successful treatment with indomethacin. *Kidney Int.* 9:302–307, 1976.
253. Zusman R.M., Keiser H.R.: Prostaglandin biosynthesis by rabbit renomedullary interstitial cells in tissue culture. *J. Clin. Invest.* 60:215–223, 1977.
254. Campbell W.B., Holland O.B., Adams B.V., et al.: Urinary excretion of prostaglandin E$_2$, prostaglandin F$_2$-alpha, and thromboxane B$_2$ in normotensive and hypertensive subjects on varying sodium intakes. *Hypertension* 4:735–741, 1982.
255. Lebel M., Grose J.H.: Renal prostaglandins in borderline and sustained essential hypertension. *Prostaglandins-Leukotrienes-Med.* 8(5):409–418, 1982.
256. Ruilope L., Garcia-Robles R., Barrietos A., et al.: The role of urinary PGE$_2$ and renin-angiotensin-aldosterone system in the pathogenesis of essential hypertension. *Clin. Exp. Hypertens.* 4(6):989–1000, 1982.
257. Sato M., Abe K., Haruyama T., et al.: Effect of dietary sodium intake on the metabolism of prostaglandins in the kidney in hypertensive patients. *Prostaglandins-Leukotrienes-Med.* 8(3):199–219, 1982.
258. Rathaus M., Bernheim J.: Effect of propranolol treatment on the urinary excretion of prostaglandins E$_2$ and F$_2$-alpha in patients with essential hypertension. *Isr. J. Med. Sci.* 18:231–234, 1982.

259. Willis L.R., Ludens J.H., Hook J.B., et al.: Mechanism of natriuretic action of bradykinin. *Am. J. Physiol.* 217:1–5, 1969.
260. Stein J.H., Congbalay R.C., Karsh D.L., et al.: The effect of bradykinin on proximal tubular sodium reabsorption in the dog: Evidence for functional nephron heterogeneity. *J. Clin. Invest.* 51:1709–1721, 1972.
261. Pierce J.V., Webster M.E.: Human plasma kallidins: Isolation and chemical studies. *Biochem. Biophys. Res. Commun.* 5:353–357, 1961.
262. Coleman R.W.: Formation of human plasma kinin. *N. Engl. J. Med.* 291:509–515, 1974.
263. Ward P.E., Gedney C.D., Dowben R.M., et al.: Isolation of membrane bound renal kallikrein and kininase. *Biochem. J.* 151:755–758, 1975.
264. Orstavik T.B., Nustad K., Brandtzaeg P., et al.: Cellular origin of urinary kallikreins. *J. Histochem. Cytochem.* 245:1037–1039, 1976.
265. Nasjletti A., Colina-Chourio J., McGiff J.C.: Disappearance of bradykinin in the renal circulation of dogs. Effect of kininase inhibition. *Circ. Res.* 37:59–65, 1975.
266. Carone F.A., Pullman T.N., Oparil S., et al.: Micropuncture evidence of rapid hydrolysis of bradykinin by rat proximal tubule. *Am. J. Physiol.* 230:1420–1424, 1976.
267. Margolius H.S., Horwitz D., Pisano J.J., et al.: Urinary kallikrein excretion in hypertensive man. Relationships to sodium intake and sodium-retaining steroids. *Circ. Res.* 35:820–825, 1974.
268. Streeten D.H.P., Kerr L.P., Kerr C.B., et al.: Hyperbradykininism: a new orthostatic syndrome. *Lancet* 2:1048–1053, 1972.
269. Wong P.Y., Talamo R.C., Williams G.H., et al.: Response of the kallikrein-kinin and renin-angiotensin systems to saline infusion and upright posture. *J. Clin. Invest.* 55:691–698, 1975.
270. Mersey J.H., Williams G.H., Hollenberg N.K., et al.: Relationship between aldosterone and bradykinin. *Circ. Res.* 40(Suppl. I):184–188, 1977.
271. Vinci J.M., Zusman R.M., Izzo J.L., et al.: Human urinary and plasma kinins. Relationship to sodium-retaining steroids and plasma renin activity. *Circ. Res.* 44(2):228–237, 1979.
272. Vane J.R., McGiff J.C.: Possible contributions of endogenous prostaglandins to the control of blood pressure. *Circ. Res.* 36–37 (Suppl. I):I-68–I-75, 1975.
273. Hong S.L., Levine L.: Stimulation of prostaglandin synthesis by bradykinin and thrombin and their mechanisms of action on MC5-5 fibroblasts. *J. Biol. Chem.* 251:5814–5816, 1976.
274. Damas J., Bourdon V.: Liberation dácide arachidonique par la bradykinine. *Comptes Rendus des Seances de la Societe de Biologie et de ses Filiales* 168:1445–1448, 1974.
275. Wong P.Y-K., Terragno D.A., Terragno N.A., et al.: Dual effects of bradykinin on prostaglandin metabolism: relationship to the dissimilar vascular actions of kinins. *Prostaglandins* 13:1113–1125, 1977.
276. Messina E.J., Weiner R., Kaley G.: Inhibition of bradykinin vasodilation and potentiation of norepinephrine and angiotensin vasoconstriction by inhibitors of prostaglandin synthesis in rat skeletal muscle. *Circ. Res.* 37:430–437, 1975.
277. McGiff J.C., Itskovitz H.D., Terragno N.A.: The action of bradykinin and

eledoisin in the canine isolated kidney; relationships to prostaglandins. *Clin. Sci.* 49:125–131, 1975.

278. Beilin L.J., Bhattacharya J.: The effects of prostaglandin synthesis inhibitors on renal blood flow distribution in conscious rabbits. *J. Physiol.* 269:395–405, 1977.

279. Terragno N.A., Terragno D.A., Pacholczyk D., et al.: Prostaglandins and the regulation of uterine blood flow in pregnancy. *Nature* 249:57–58, 1974.

280. Erdos E.G.: The kinins. A status report. *Biochem. Pharmacol.* 25:1563–1569, 1976.

281. Erdos E.G.: Angiotensin I converting enzyme. *Circ. Res.* 36:247–255, 1975.

282. McGiff J.C., Terragno N.A., Malik K.U., et al.: Release of a prostaglandin E-like substance from canine kidney by bradykinin. *Circ. Res.* 31:36–43, 1972.

283. Margolius H.S., Geller R., de Jong W., et al.: Altered urinary kallikrein excretion in rats with hypertension. *Circ. Res.* 30:358–362, 1972.

284. Elliot A.H., Nuzum F.R.: Urinary excretion of a depressor substance (kallikrein of Frey and Kraut) in arterial hypertension. *Endocrinology* 18:462–474, 1934.

285. Bevan V.H., Pierce J.V., Pisano J.J.: A sensitive isotopic procedure for the assay of esterase activity: Measurement of human urinary kallikrein. *Clin. Chem. Acta* 32:67–73, 1971.

286. Levy S.B., Lilley J.J., Frigon R.P., et al.: Urinary kallikrein and plasma renin activity as determinants of renal blood flow; the influence of race and dietary sodium intake. *J. Clin. Invest.* 60:129–138, 1977.

287. Zinner S.H., Margolius H.S., Rosner B., et al.: Eight year longitudinal study of blood pressure and urinary kallikrein in childhood. *Clin. Res.* 25:266A, 1977.

288. Nasjletti A., Colina-Chourio J.: Interaction of mineralocorticoids, renal prostaglandins and the renal kallikrein-kinin system. *Fed. Proc.* 35:189–193, 1976.

289. Keiser H.R., Andrews M.J. Jr., Guyton R.A., et al.: Urinary kallikrein in dogs with constriction of one renal artery. *Proc. Soc. Exp. Biol. Med.* 151:53–56, 1976.

290. Mills I.H., MacFarlane N.A.A., Ward P.E.: The renal kallikrein-kinin system and the regulation of salt and water excretion. *Fed. Proc.* 35:181–188, 1976.

291. Hulthén U.L., Lecerof H., Hokfelt B.: Renal venous output of kinins in patients with hypertension and unilateral renal artery stenosis. *Acta Med. Scand.* 202:189–191, 1977.

292. Zinner S.H., Margolius H.S., Rosner B., et al.: Familial aggregation of urinary kallikrein concentration in childhood: relation to blood pressure, race and urinary electrolytes. *Am. J. Epidemiol.* 104:124–132, 1976.

293. O'Connor D.T.: Response of the renal kallikrein-kinin system, intravascular volume, and renal hemodynamics to sodium restriction and diuretic treatment in essential hypertension. *Hypertension* 4(Suppl. III):III-72–III-78, 1982.

294. O'Connor D.T., Bars A.P., Amend W., et al.: Urinary kallikrein excretion after renal transplantation: Relationship to hypertension, graft source, and renal function. *Am. J. Med.* 73(4):475–481, 1982.

295. Saruta T., Kondo K.: Endocrine factors in juvenile essential hypertension. *Jpn. J. Med.* 21(2):152–154, 1982.
296. Margolius H.S., Horwitz D., Pisano J.J., et al.: Relationships among urinary kallikrein, mineralocorticoids and human hypertensive disease. *Fed. Proc.* 35:203–206, 1976.
297. Galvez O.G., Bay W.H., Roberts B.W., et al.: The hemodynamic effects of potassium deficiency in the dog. *Circ. Res.* 40:I-11–I-16, 1977.
298. McGiff J.C.: Bartter's syndrome results from an imbalance of vasoactive hormones. *Ann. Intern. Med.* 87:369–372, 1977.
299. Vinci J., Zusman R., Bowden R., et al.: Relationship of urinary and plasma kinins to sodium-retaining steroids and plasma renin activity. *Clin. Res.* 25:450A, 1977.
300. Marin-Grez M., Cottone P., Carretero A.: Evidence for an involvement of kinins in regulation of sodium excretion. *Am. J. Physiol.* 223:794–796, 1972.
301. Nasjletti A., McGiff J.C., Colina-Chourio J.: Interrelationships of the renal kallikrein-kinin and prostaglandin systems in the conscious rat: Influence of mineralocorticoids. *Circ. Res.* 43:799–807, 1978.
302. Marin-Grez M.: The influence of antibodies against bradykinin on isotonic saline diuresis in the rat. *Pflugers Arch.* 350:231–239, 1974.
303. Colina-Chourio J., McGiff J.C., Miller M.P., et al.: Possible influence of intrarenal generation of kinins on prostaglandin release from the rabbit perfused kidney. *Br. J. Pharmacol.* 58:165–172, 1976.
304. Carretero O.A., Scicli A.G.: Renal kallikrein: its localization and possible role in renal function. *Fed. Proc.* 35:194–198, 1976.
305. Weber P.C., Larsson C., Scherer B.: Prostaglandin E_2-9-ketoreductase as a mediator of salt intake-related prostaglandin-renin interaction. *Nature* 266:65–66, 1977.
306. O'Connor D.T.: Response of the renal kallikrein-kinin system, intravascular volume, and renal hemodynamics to sodium restriction and diuretic treatment in essential hypertension. *Hypertension* 4(2):II-172–177, 1982.
307. Muirhead E.E.: Antihypertensive functions of the kidney. *Hypertension* 2:444–464, 1980.
308. Muirhead E.E., Stirman J.A., Jones F.: Renal autotransplantation and protection against renoprival hypertensive cardiovascular disease and hemolysis. *J. Clin. Invest.* 39:266–281, 1960.
309. Muirhead E.E., Rightsel W.A., Leach B.E., et al.: Reversal of hypertension by transplants and lipid extracts of cultured renomedullary interstitial cells. *Lab. Invest.* 36:162–172, 1977.
310. Tobian L., Azar S.: Antihypertensive and other functions of the renal papilla. *Trans. Assoc. Am. Physicians* 84:281–288, 1971.
311. Manthorpe T.: Antihypertensive and hypertensive effects of the kidney. *Acta Pathol. Microbiol. Immunol. Scand.* 83A:395–405, 1975.
312. Susic D., Sparks J.C., Machado E.A., et al.: The mechanisms of renomedullary antihypertensive action, haemodynamic studies in hydronephrotic rats with one-clip hypertension. *Clin. Sci. Mol. Med.* 54:361–367, 1978.
313. Gothberg G., Lundin S., Folkow B.: Acute vasodepressor effect in normotensive rats following extracorporeal perfusion of the declipped kidney of two-kidney, one-clip hypertensive rats. *Hypertension* 4(suppl. II):II-101–II-105, 1982.

314. Muirhead E.E., Folkow B., Byers L.W., et al.: Cardiovascular effects of antihypertensive polar and neutral renomedullary lipids. *Hypertension* 5(suppl I):I-112–I-118, 1983.
315. Faber J.E., Barron K.W., Bonham A.C., et al.: Regional hemodynamic effects of antihypertensive renomedullary lipids in conscious rats. *Hypertension* 6:494–502, 1984.
316. Muirhead E.E.: Case for a renomedullary blood pressure lowering hormone, in Eisenbach G.M., Brod J. (eds.): *Contributions to Nephrology*, Vol. 12. Basel, S. Karger A.G., 1978, pp. 69–81.
317. Edmondson R., Hilton P., Jones W.: Abnormal leucocyte composition and sodium transport in essential hypertension. *Lancet* 1:1003–1005, 1975.
318. Garay R.P., Elghozi J.L., Gagher G., et al.: Laboratory distinction between essential and secondary hypertension by measurement of erythrocyte cation fluxes. *N. Engl. J. Med.* 302:769–771, 1980.
319. Ghione S., Buzzigoli G., Bartolini V., et al.: Comparison of outward and inward $Na+/K+$ cotransport-mediated fluxes in erythrocytes in essential hypertensive patients. Preliminary results. *Clin. Exp. Hypertens.* 3(4):809–814, 1981.
320. Cusi O., Barlassina C., Ferrandi M., et al.: Familial aggregation of cation transport abnormalities and essential hypertension. *Clin. Exp. Hypertension* 3(4):871–884, 1981.
321. Swarts H.G., Bonting S.L., de Pont J., et al.: Cation fluxes in $Na+-K+-$activated ATPase activity in erythrocytes of patients with essential hypertension. *Hypertension* 3:641–649, 1981.
322. Walter U., Distler A.: Abnormal sodium efflux in erythrocytes of patients with essential hypertension. *Hypertension* 4:205–210, 1982.
323. Duhm J., Gobel O.B., Lorenz R., et al.: Sodium-lithium exchange and sodium-potassium cotransport in human erythrocytes. Part 2: A simple uptake test applied to normotensive and essential hypertensive individuals. *Hypertension* 4:477–482, 1982.
324. Adragna N.C., Canessa M.L., Solomon H., et al.: Red cell lithium-sodium countertransport and sodium-potassium cotransport in patients with essential hypertension. *Hypertension* 4:795–804, 1982.
325. Tuck M.L., Gross C., Maxwell M., et al.: Erythrocyte $Na+$, $K+$ cotransport and $Na+$, $K+$ pump in black and caucasian hypertensive patients. *Hypertension* 6:536–544, 1984.
326. Canessa M.N., Adragna N., Soloman H.S., et al.: Increased sodium-lithium counter-transport in red cells of patients with essential hypertension. *N. Engl. J. Med.* 302:772–776, 1980.
327. Woods J.W., Falk R.J., Pittman A.W., et al.: Increased red-cell sodium-lithium countertransport in normotensive sons of hypertensive parents. *N. Engl. J. Med.* 306:593–595, 1982.
328. Trevisan M., Ostrow D., Cooper R., et al.: Abnormal red cell ion transport and hypertension. The People's Gas Study. *Hypertension* 5:363–367, 1983.
329. Brugnara C., Corrocher R., Foroni L., et al.: Lithium-sodium countertransport in erythrocytes of normal and hypertensive subjects. *Hypertension* 5:529–534, 1983.
330. Duhm J., Gobel O.B.: Sodium-lithium exchange and sodium-potassium

cotransport in human erythrocytes. Part 1: Evaluation of a simple uptake test to assess the activity of the two transport systems. *Hypertension* 4:468–476, 1982.

331. Isben K.K., Jensen H.E., Wieth J.O., et al.: Sodium-lithium countertransport in erythrocytes from patients and from children having one hypertensive parent. *Hypertension* 4:703–709, 1982.

332. Chesley L.C.: The origin of the word "eclampsia." A vindication of deSauvages. *Obstet. Gynecol.* 39:802–804, 1972.

333. Castelli B.: Castellus Renovatus: Hoc. Est. *Lexicon Medicum, quondam a Barth,* Norimbergae, Tauberi J.D., 1682.

334. deSauvages F.B.S.: *Pathologia Methodica, seu de Cognescendis Morbis,* ed. 3. Leyden, Fratum de Tournes, 1759, p. 286.

335. *Stedman's Medical Dictionary 1957 (ed. 19), 1961 (ed. 20),* Baltimore, Williams & Wilkins Co. p. 1449.

336. Gant N.F., Hutchinson H.T., Siiteri P.K., et al.; Study of the metabolic clearance rate of dehydroisoandrosterone sulfate in pregnancy. *Am. J. Obstet. Gynecol.* 111:555–563, 1971.

337. Lunell N.O., Nylund L.E., Lewander R., et al.: Uteroplacental blood flow in preeclampsia measurements with indium 113m and a computer-linked gamma camera. *Clin. Exp. Hypertens.* 1:105–117, 1982.

338. Page E.W.: On the pathogenesis of preeclampsia and eclampsia. *J. Obstet. Gynaecol. Br. Commonw.* 79:883–894, 1972.

339. Senior J.B., Fahim I., Sullivan F.M., et al.: Possible role of 5-hydroxytryptamine in toxemia of pregnancy. *Lancet* 2:553–554, 1963.

340. Sandler M., Baldock E.: In vivo monoamine oxidase activity in toxemia of pregnancy. *J. Obstet. Gynaecol. Br. Commonw.* 70:279–283, 1963.

341. Werkö L.: Studies in the problems of circulation in pregnancy, in Hammond J., Browne F.J., Wolsterholme G.E.W. (eds.): *Toxaemias of Pregnancy. Ciba Foundation Symposium.* London, Churchill, 1950, p. 155.

342. Burt C.C.: Forearm and hand blood flow in pregnancy, in Hammond J., Browne F.J., Wolsterhome G.E.W. (eds.): *Toxemias of Pregnancy. Ciba Foundation Symposium.* London, Churchill-Livingstone, 1950, p. 151.

343. Munnell E.W., Taylor H.C. Jr.: Liver blood flow in pregnancy-hepatic vein catheterization. *J. Clin. Invest.* 26:952–956, 1947.

344. Bucht H., Werkö L.: Glomerular filtration rate on renal blood flow in hypertensive toxemia of pregnancy. *J. Obstet. Gynaec. Br. Emp.* 60:157–164, 1953.

345. Browne J.C.M., Veall N.: The maternal placental blood flow in normotensive and hypertensive women. *J. Obstet. Gynaecol. Br. Emp.* 60:141–147, 1953.

346. White R.: Symposium on haemodynamics in pregnancy. III. Blood volume in pregnancy. *Trans. Edinb. Obstet. Soc.* 57:14–17, 1950.

347. Werkö L., Brody S.: The blood-pressure in toxaemia of pregnancy. I. Spontaneous diurnal variability. *J. Obstet. Gynaecol. Br. Emp.* 60:180–185, 1953.

348. Smith S.L., Douglas B.H., Langford H.G.: A model of preeclampsia. *Johns Hopkins Med. J.* 120:220–224, 1967.

349. Carlsson C.: Cardiovascular changes in preeclampsia. *Acta Obstet. Gynecol. Scand.* 118:121–122, 1984.

350. Kúzniar J., Piela A., Skret A., et al.: Echocardiographic estimation of hemodynamics in hypertensive pregnancy. *Am. J. Obstet. Gynecol.* 144:430–470, 1982.

351. Kúzniar J., Piela A., Skret A.: Left ventricular function in preeclamptic patients: an echocardiographic study. *Am. J. Obstet. Gynecol.* 146(4):400–405, 1983.

352. Phelan J.P., Yurth D.A.: Severe preeclampsia. I. Peripartum hemodynamic observations. *Am. J. Obstet. Gynecol.* 144:17–22, 1982.

353. Dieckmann W.J., Machel H.L., Woodruff P.W.: The cold pressor test in pregnancy. *Am. J. Obstet. Gynecol.* 36:408–412, 1938.

354. Browne F.J.: The cold pressor test in pregnancy. *J. Obstet. Gynaecol. Br. Emp.* 47:365–370, 1940.

355. Raab W., Schroeder G., Wagner R., et al.: Vascular reactivity and electrolytes in normal and toxemic pregnancy. *J. Clin. Endocrinol. Metab.* 16:1196–1216, 1956.

356. Zuspan F.P., Nelson G.H., Ahlquist R.P.: Epinephrine infusions in normal and toxemic pregnancy. *Am. J. Obstet. Gynecol.* 90:88–98, 1964.

357. Chesley L.C., Talledo E., Bohler C.S., et al.: Vascular reactivity to angiotensin II and norepinephrine in pregnant and nonpregnant women. *Am. J. Obstet. Gynecol.* 91:837–842, 1965.

358. Abdul-Karim R., Assali N.S.: Pressor response to angiotensin in pregnant and nonpregnant women. *Am. J. Obstet. Gynecol.* 82:246–251, 1961.

359. Kaplan N.M., Silah J.G.: Effect of angiotensin II on the blood pressure in humans with hypertensive disease. *J. Clin. Invest.* 43:659–669, 1964.

360. Hocken A.G., Kark R.M., Passavoy M.: Angiotensin infusion test. *Lancet* 1:5–10, 1966.

361. Chesley L.C., Tepper I.H.: Effects of progesterone and estrogen on the sensitivity to angiotensin II. *J. Chem. Endocrinol.* 27:576–581, 1967.

362. Morandini G., Mangioni C.: La resposta pressoria all angiotensia e alla noradrenalina nella gravidanza normale enella sindrome gestosica. *Minerva Med.* 58:1546–1552, 1967.

363. Talledo O.E., Chesley L.C., Zuspan F.P.: Renin-angiotensin system in normal and toxemic pregnancies. *Am. J. Obstet. Gynecol.* 100:218–221, 1968.

364. Mendlowitz M., Aletchek A., Naftchi N., et al.: Digital vascular reactivity to L-norepinephrine in the second trimester of pregnancy as a test for latent essential hypertension and toxemia. *Am. J. Obstet. Gynecol.* 81:643–652, 1961.

365. Dieckmann W.J., Michel H.L.: Vascular effects of posterior pituitary extracts in pregnant women. *Am. J. Obstet. Gynecol.* 33:131–137, 1937.

366. Browne F.J.; Sensitization of the vascular system in preeclamptic toxemia and eclampsia. *J. Obstet. Gynaecol. Br. Emp.* 53:510–518, 1946.

367. Brust A.A., Assali N.S., Ferris E.B.: Evaluation of neurogenic and humoral factors in blood pressure maintenance in normal and toxemic pregnancy using tetraethylammonium chloride. *J. Clin. Invest.* 27:717–726, 1948.

368. Chesley L.C.: Vascular reactivity in normal and toxemic pregnancy. *Clin. Obstet. Gynecol.* 9:871–881, 1966.

369. Assali N.S., Prystowsky H.: Studies on autonomic blockade. *J. Clin. Invest.* 29:1354–1366, 1950.

370. Sims E.A.H.: The kidney in pregnancy, in Strauss M.B., Welt L.C. (eds.): *Diseases of the Kidney*, ed. 2. Boston, Little, Brown & Co., 1971, p. 1155.
371. Bucht H.: Studies on renal function in man with special reference to glomerular filtration and renal plasma flow in pregnancy. *J. Clin. Lab. Invest.* 3 (Suppl 3):1–64, 1951.
372. Levitt M.F.: Clinical conference on medical hazards of pregnancy. *J. Mt. Sinai Hosp.* 24:472–498, 1957.
373. Sims E.A.H., Krantz K.E.: Serial studies of renal function during pregnancy and the puerperium in normal women. *J. Clin. Invest.* 37:1764–1774, 1958.
374. Chesley L.C., Sloan D.M.: The effect of posture on renal function in late pregnancy. *Am. J. Obstet. Gynecol.* 89:754–759, 1964.
375. Assali N.S., Dignam W.J., Dasgupta K.: Renal function in human pregnancy. II. The effects of venous pooling on renal hemodynamics and water, electrolyte, and aldosterone excretion during normal gestation. *J. Lab. Clin. Med.* 54:394–408, 1959.
376. Pritchard J.A., Barnes A.C., Bright R.H.: The effect of the supine position on renal function in the near-term pregnant woman. *J. Clin. Invest.* 34:777–781, 1955.
377. Baird D.T., Gasson P.W., Doig A.: The renogram in pregnancy with particular reference to changes produced by alteration in posture. *Am. J. Obstet. Gynecol.* 95:597–603, 1966.
378. Crabtree E.G.: *Urological Diseases of Pregnancy.* Boston, Little, Brown & Co., 1942.
379. Fainstat F.: Ureteral dilatation of pregnancy: A review. *Obstet. Gynecol. Surv.* 18:845–860, 1963.
380. Traut H.F., McLane C.M.: Physiological changes in ureter associated with pregnancy. *Surg. Gynecol. Obstet.* 62:65–72, 1936.
381. Kalousek G., Hlavacek C., Nedoss B., et al.: Circadian rhythms of creatinine and electrolyte excretion in healthy pregnant women. *Am. J. Obstet. Gynecol.* 103:856–867, 1969.
382. Rosenthal H.E., Slaunwhite W.R. Jr., Sandberg A.A.: Transcortin: A corticosteroid-binding protein of plasma. X. Cortisol and progesterone interplay and unbound levels of these steroids in pregnancy. *J. Clin. Endocrinol. Metab.* 29:352–367, 1969.
383. Landau R.L., Lugibihl K.: Inhibition of the sodium-retaining influence of aldosterone by progesterone. *J. Clin. Endocrinol. Metab.* 18:1237–1245, 1958.
384. Beyers A.D., Odendaal H.J., Spruyt L.L., et al.: The possible role of endogenous digitalis-like substance in the causation of preeclampsia. *S. Afr. Med. J.* 65:883–885, 1984.
385. Löhlein M.: Zur Pathogenese der Nierenkrankheiten II. Nephritis und Nephrose, mit besonderer Berucksichtigung der Nephropathia gravidarium. *Deutsche Med. Wochenschr.* 44:851–1187, 1918.
386. Spargo B., McCartney C.P., Winemiller R.: Glomerular capillary endotheliosis in toxemia in pregnancy. *Arch. Pathol. Lab. Med.* 68:593–599, 1959.
387. Pollack V.E., Nettles J.B.: The kidney in toxemia of pregnancy: A clinical and pathological study based on renal biopsies. *Medicine* 39:469–526, 1960.
388. Altchek S., Albright N.L., Somers S.C.; The renal pathology of toxemia of pregnancy. *Obstet. Gynecol.* 31:595–607, 1968.

389. Altchek A.: Electron microscopy of renal biopsies in toxemia of pregnancy. *J.A.M.A.* 175:791–795, 1961.
390. McCartney C.P., Spargo B., Larincz A.B., et al.: Renal structure and function in pregnant patients with acute hypertension. *Am. J. Obstet. Gynecol.* 90:579–592, 1964.
391. Sarles H.E., Hill S.S., LeBlanc A.L., et al.: Sodium excretion patterns during the following intravenous sodium chloride loads in normal and hypertensive pregnancies. *Am. J. Obstet. Gynecol.* 102:1–7, 1968.
392. Bucht H., Werkö L.: Glomerular filtration rate and renal blood flow in hypertensive toxaemia of pregnancy. *J. Obstet. Gynaecol. Br. Emp.* 60:157–164, 1953.
393. Smith H.W.: *The Kidney-Structure and Function in Health and Disease.* New York, Oxford University Press, 1951.
394. Assali N.S., Kaplan S.A., Fomon S.J., et al.: Renal function studies in toxemia of pregnancy. *J. Clin. Invest.* 32:44–51, 1953.
395. Little B.: Water and electrolyte balance during pregnancy. *Anesthesiology* 26:400–408, 1965.
396. Redd J., Mosel L.M., Langford H.G.: Effect of posture upon sodium excretion in preeclampsia. *Am. J. Obstet. Gynecol.* 100:343–347, 1968.
397. Preedy J.R.K., Aitken E.H.: Plasma oestrogen levels in late pregnancy, in the normal menstruating female, and in the male. *Lancet* 1:191–192, 1957.
398. Fishman J., Brown J.B., Hellman L., et al.: Estrogen metabolism in normal and pregnant women. *J. Biol. Chem.* 237:1489–1494, 1962.
399. Dignam W.S., Vaskian J., Assali N.S.: Effects of estrogens on renal hemodynamics and excretion of electrolytes in human subjects. *J. Clin. Endocrinol. Metab.* 16:1032–1042, 1956.
400. Helmer O.M., Judson W.E.: Influence of high renin substrate levels on renin-angiotensin system in pregnancy. *Am. J. Obstet. Gynecol.* 99:9–17, 1967.
401. Laragh J.H.: High blood pressure and oral contraceptives. Changes in plasma renin and renin substrate and in aldosterone excretion. *Am. J. Obstet. Gynecol.* 101:1037–1045, 1968.
402. Shearman R.P.: Some aspects of the urinary excretion of pregnanediol pregnancy. *J. Obstet. Gynaecol. Br. Commonw.* 66:1–11, 1959.
403. Devis R.: Elimination of corticoids during pregnancy. *Gynecol. Obstet.* (Paris) 53:57–77, 1954.
404. Tobian L. Jr.: Corticol steroid excretion in edema of pregnancy, preeclampsia, and essential hypertension. *J. Clin. Endocrinol. Metab.* 9:319–329, 1949.
405. Parvianinen S., Soiva K., Vartianen S.: Corticosteroid excretion during pregnancy, especially in toxaemia of late pregnancy. *Acta Obstet. Gynecol. Scand.* 29(Suppl 5):1–17, 1950.
406. Appleby J.I., Norymberski J.K.: The urinary excretion of 17 hydroxycorticosteroids in human pregnancy. *J. Endocrinol.* 15:310–319, 1957.
407. Huis in 't Veld L.G.: Excretion of 17-ketosteroids during pregnancy. *Gynecol. Obstet.* (Paris) 53:42–56, 1954.
408. Martin J.D., Mills I.H.: Aldosterone excretion in normal and toxaemic pregnancies. *Br. Med. J.* 2:571–573, 1956.
409. O'Connell M., Welsh G.W. III: Unbound plasma cortisol in pregnant and

enovid-E-treated women as determined by ultrafiltration. *J. Clin. Endocrinol. Metab.* 29:563–568, 1959.

410. Kopelman J.J., Levitz M.: Plasma cortisol levels and cortisol binding in normal and preeclamptic pregnancies. *Am. J. Obstet. Gynecol.* 108:925–930, 1970.

411. Bromberg Y.M., Sadowsky A., Shulman F.G.: Corticotropin in blood in pregnancy. *J.A.M.A.* 154:165, 1954.

412. Hunt A.B., McConakey W.M.: Pregnancy associated with diseases of adrenal glands. *Am. J. Obstet. Gynecol.* 66:970–987, 1953.

413. Shizume K., Lerner A.B.: Determination of melanocyte-stimulating hormone in urine and blood. *J. Clin. Endocrinol. Metab.* 14:1491–1510, 1954.

414. Dowling J.T., Freinkel N., Ingbar S.H.: Thyroxine-binding by sera of pregnant women. *J. Clin. Endocrinol. Metab.* 16:280–282, 1956.

415. Diczfalusey D.: Chorionic gonadotropin and oestrogens in human placenta. *Acta Endocrinol.* (Copenh) (Suppl. 12), 1953, pp. 9–175.

416. Kaplan S.L., Brumback M.M.: Studies of a human and simian placental hormone with growth hormone-like and prolactin-like activities. *J. Clin. Endocrinol. Metab.* 24:80–100, 1964.

417. Del Greco F., Krumlovskey F.A.: The renal pressor system in human pregnancy. *J. Reprod. Med.* 8:98–101, 1972.

418. Ehrlich E.N., Lindheimer M.D.: Sodium metabolism, aldosterone, and the hypertensive disorders of pregnancy. *J. Reprod. Med.* 8:106–110, 1972.

419. Kokot F., Cekanski A.: Plasma renin activity in peripheral and uterine vein blood in pregnant and nonpregnant women. *J. Obstet. Gynaecol. Br. Commonw.* 79:72–76, 1972.

420. Weir R.J., Paintin D.B., Brown J.J., et al.: A serial study in pregnancy of the plasma concentrations of renin, cortico-steroids, electrolytes, and proteins. *J. Obstet. Gynaecol. Br. Commonw.* 78:590–602, 1971.

421. Gordon R.D., Parsons S., Symonds C.M.: A prospective study of plasma renin activity in normal and toxemic pregnancy. *Lancet* 1:347–349, 1969.

422. Massani Z.M., Sanguinett R., Gallegos R., et al.: Angiotensin blood levels in normal and toxemic pregnancies. *Am. J. Obstet. Gynecol.* 99:313–317, 1967.

423. Boonshaft B., O'Connell J.M.B., Hayes J.M., et al.: Serum renin activity during normal pregnancy. *J. Clin. Endocrinol.* 28:1641–1644, 1968.

424. Gordon R.D., Fishman L.M., Liddle G.W.: Plasma renin activity and aldosterone secretion in a pregnant woman with primary aldosteronism. *J. Clin. Endocrinol.* 27:385–388, 1967.

425. Gould A.B., Skeggs L.T., Kahn J.R.: Measurement of renin and substrate concentration in human serum. *Lab. Invest.* 15:1802–1813, 1966.

426. Maebashi M., Aida M., Yoshinaga K., et al.: Estimation of circulatory renin in normal and toxemic pregnancy. *Tohoku J. Exp. Med.* 84:55–61, 1965.

427. Brown J.J., Davies D.L., Doak P.B., et al.: Serial estimation of plasma renin concentration during pregnancy and after parturition, *J. Endocrinol.* 35:373–378, 1966.

428. Skinner S.L., Lumbers E.R., Symonds E.M.: Renin concentration in human fetal and maternal tissues. *Am. J. Obstet. Gynecol.* 101:529–533, 1968.

429. Laragh J.H.: The pill, hypertension and the toxemias of pregnancy. *Am. J. Obstet. Gynecol.* 109:210–213, 1971.

430. Saruta T., Saade G., Kaplan N.M.; A possible mechanism for hypertension induced by oral contraceptives. *Arch. Intern. Med.* 126:621–626, 1970.
431. Crane M.G., Harris J.J., Windsor W. III: Hypertension, oral contraceptive agents and conjugated estrogens. *Ann. Intern. Med.* 74:13–21, 1971.
432. Newton M.A., Sealey J.E., Ledingham S.C.G., et al.: High blood pressure and oral contraceptives. *Am. J. Obstet. Gynecol.* 101:1037–1045, 1968.
433. Jones K.M., Lloyd-Jones R., Riondel A., et al.: Aldosterone secretion and metabolism in normal men and women in pregnancy. *Acta Endocrinol.* 30:321–342, 1959.
434. Watanabe M., Meeker M.L., Gray M.J., et al.: Secretion of aldosterone in normal pregnancy. *J. Clin. Invest.* 42:1619–1631, 1963.
435. Ehrlich E.N., Lindheimer M.D.: Effect of administered mineralocorticoids or ACTH in pregnant women. Attenuation of kaliuretic influence of mineralocorticoids during pregnancy. *J. Clin. Invest.* 51:1301–1309, 1972.
436. Biglieri E.G., Slaton P.E., Kronfield S.J., et al.: Diagnosis of an aldosterone-producing adenoma in primary aldosteronism. An evaluative maneuver. *J.A.M.A.* 201:510–514, 1967.
437. Ehrlich E.N., Laves M., Landau R.I.: Progesterone-aldosterone interrelationships in pregnancy. *J. Lab. Clin. Med.* 59:588–595, 1962.
438. Boonshaft B., O'Connell J.M.B., Hayes J.M. et al.: Serum renin activity during normal pregnancy: Effect of alterations of posture and sodium intake. *J. Clin. Endocrinol. Metab.* 28:1641–1644, 1968.
439. Ehrlich E.N., Lugibihl K., Taylor C., et al.: Reciprocal variations in urinary cortisol and aldosterone in response to the sodium-depleting influence of hydrochlorothiazide and ethacrynic acid in humans. *J. Clin. Endocrinol. Metab.* 27:836–842, 1967.
440. Ehrlich E.N.: Heparinoid-induced inhibition of aldosterone secretion in normal pregnant women. The rate of augmented aldosterone secretion in sodium conservation during normal pregnancy. *Am. J. Obstet. Gynecol.* 109:963–970, 1971.
441. Gordon E.S., Chart J.J., Hayedaen D., et al.: Mechanisms of sodium retention in preeclamptic toxemia. *Obstet. Gynecol.* 4:39–50, 1954.
442. Vande Wiele R.L., Gurpide E., Kelley W.G., et al.: The secretory rate of progesterone and aldosterone in normal and abnormal late pregnancy. *Acta Endocrinol.* 35(Suppl. 51):159, 1960.
443. Watanabe M., Murker C.L., Gray M.J., et al.: Aldosterone secretion rates in abnormal pregnancy. *J. Clin. Endocrinol. Metab.* 25:1665–1670, 1965.
444. Moses A.M., Lobatsky J., Lloyd C.W.: The occurrence of pre-eclampsia in a bilaterally adrenalectomized woman. *J. Clin. Endocrinol. Metab.* 19:987–994, 1959.
445. Smith G.V., Smith O.W.: Estrogen and progestin metabolism in pregnant women, with special reference to pre-eclamptic toxemia and the effect of hormone administration. *Am. J. Obstet. Gynecol.* 39:405–422, 1940.
446. Strand A.: The function of the placenta and "placental insufficiency" with especial reference to the development of prolonged fetal distress. *Acta Obstet. Gynecol. Scand.* 28:426–445, 1949.
447. Frandsen V.A., Stakemann G.: Urinary excretion of estriol during normal pregnancy. *Dan. Med. Bull.* 7:95–98, 1960.
448. Coyle M.G., Greig M., Walker J.: Blood-progesterone and urinary preg-

nanediol and oestrogens in fetal death from severe pre-eclampsia. *Lancet* 2:275–277, 1962.

449. Bonar J., Brown J.J., Davies D.L., et al.: Plasma renin concentration in American Negro women with hypertensive disease of pregnancy. *J. Obstet. Gynaecol. Br. Commonw.* 73:418–420, 1966.

450. Hodari A.A.: Chronic uterine ischemia and reversable experimental "toxemia of pregnancy." *Am. J. Obstet. Gynecol.* 97:597–607, 1967.

451. Hodari A.A., Bumpus F.M., Smedby R.: Renin in experimental "toxemia of pregnancy." *Obstet. Gynecol.* 30:8–15, 1967.

452. Hodari A.A.: The contribution of the fetal kidney to experimental hypertensive disease of pregnancy. *Am. J. Obstet. Gynecol.* 101:17–22, 1968.

453. Hodari A.A., Hodgkinson C.P.: Fetal kidney as source of renin in the pregnant dog. *Am. J. Obstet. Gynecol.* 102:691–701, 1968.

454. Hodgkinson C.P., Hodari A.A., Bumpus F.M.: Experimental hypertensive disease in pregnancy. *Obstet. Gynecol.* 30:371–380, 1967.

455. Smith G.V., Smith O.W.: Excessive anterior-pituitary-like hormone and variations in oestrin in toxemias of late pregnancy. *Proc. Soc. Exp. Biol. Med.* 30:918–919, 1933.

456. Smith G.V., Smith O.W.: Excessive gonad-stimulating hormone and subnormal amounts of oestrin in toxemias of late pregnancy. *Am. J. Physiol.* 107:128–145, 1934.

457. Rubin B.L., Dorfman R.I., Miller M.: Hormone metabolites in blood and urine of diabetic pregnant patients with and without toxemia. *J. Clin. Endocrinol. Metab.* 6:347–368, 1946.

458. Smith G.V., Smith O.W.: Anterior pituitary-like hormone in late pregnancy toxemia; summary of results since 1932. *Am. J. Obstet. Gynecol.* 38:618–624, 1939.

459. Smith G.V., Smith O.W.: Estrogen and progestin metabolism in pregnancy; endocrine imbalance of pre-eclampsia and eclampsia. Summary of findings to Feb. 1941. *J. Clin. Endocrinol. Metab.* 1:470–476, 1941.

460. Smith O.W., Smith G.V., Hurwitz D.: Relationship between hormonal abnormalities and accidents of late pregnancy in diabetic women. *Am. J. Med. Sci.* 208:25–35, 1944.

461. Watts R.M., Adair F.L.: Excretion of estrogen and gonadotropin in late pregnancy, with especial reference to toxemias of pregnancy and to quantitative methods. *Am. J. Obstet. Gynecol.* 46:183–207, 1943.

462. Cohen H.M., Wilson D.A., Brennan W.F.: Blood gonadotropic determinations in relation to toxemia of pregnancy. *Penn. Med.* 46:1282–1285, 1943.

463. Paterson M.L.: The role of the posterior pituitary antidiuretic hormone in toxaemia of pregnancy. *J. Obstet. Gynaecol. Br. Emp.* 67:883–898, 1960.

464. Bloemers D.: Diabetes insipidus and toxaemis of pregnancy. *J. Obstet. Gynaecol. Br. Emp.* 68:322–327, 1961.

465. Sullivan J.M., McGiff J.C.: Kallikrein-Kinin and Prostaglandin-System in Hypertension, in Rosenthal J. (ed.): *Arterial Hypertension.* New York, Springer-Verlag New York, 1982, p. 170.

466. Terragno N.A., Terragno D.A., McGiff J.C.: The role of prostaglandins in the control of uterine blood flow, in Lindheimer M.D., Katz A.L., Zuspan F.D. (eds.): *Hypertension in Pregnancy.* New York, John Wiley & Sons, 1976, p. 391.

467. Bay W.H., Ferris T.F.: Factors controlling plasma renin and aldosterone during pregnancy. *Hypertension* 1(4):410–415, 1979.
468. Editorial: PG-synthetase inhibitors in obstetrics and after. *Lancet* 2:185–186, 1980.
469. Frölich J.C., Wilson T.W.: Urinary prostaglandins: Identification and origin. *J. Clin. Invest.* 55:763–770, 1975.
470. Gerber J.G., Payne N.A., Murphy R.C., et al.: Prostacyclin produced by the pregnant uterus in the dog may act as a circulating vasodepressor substance. *J. Clin. Invest.* 67:632–636, 1981.
471. Omini C., Folco G.C., Pasargiklian R., et al.: Prostacyclin in pregnant human uterus. *Prostaglandins* 17:113–119, 1979.
472. Hamberg M., Tuoemo T., Svenson J., et al.: Formation and action of prostacyclin in isolated human umbilical artery. *Acta Physiol. Scand.* 106:289–292, 1979.
473. Henrich W.L.: Role of prostaglandins in renin secretion. *Kidney Int.* 19:822–830, 1981.
474. Everett R.B., Worley R.J., MacDonald P.G., et al.: Effect of prostaglandin synthetase inhibition on pressor response to angiotensin II in human pregnancy. *J. Clin. Endocrinol. Metab.* 46:1007–1010, 1978.
475. Ferris T.F.: Toxemia and Hypertension, in Burrow G.N., Ferris T.F. (eds.): *Medical Complications During Pregnancy, ed. 2*. Philadelphia, W.B. Saunders Co., 1982, pp. 1–35.
476. Kaplan N.M.: *Clinical Hypertension, ed.3*. Baltimore, Williams & Wilkins Company, 1982, p. 367.
477. Fidler J., Bennett M.J., deSwiet M., et al.: Treatment of pregnancy hypertension with prostacyclin. (letter), *Lancet* 2:31–32, 1980.
477a. Jouppila P., Kirkinen P., Koivula A. et al.: Failure of exogenous prostacyclin to change placental and fetal blood flow in preeclampsia. *Am. J. Obstet. Gynecol.* 151:661–665, 1985.
478. Katz J., Troll W., Levy M., et al.: Estrogen-dependent trypsin-like activity in the rat uterus. *Arch. Biochem. Biophys.* 173:347–354, 1976.
479. Carretero O.A., Nasjletti A., Inon A., et al.: Kinins, kininogen, and kininogenase activity of pregnancy and hepatic failure. *Am. J. Med. Sci.* 259:182–186, 1970.
480. Valdes G., Espinosa P., Moore R., et al.: Urinary kallikrein and plasma renin activity in normal human pregnancy. *Hypertension* 3:II-55–II-58, 1981.
481. Elebute O.A., Mills I.H.: Urinary kallirein in normal and hypertensive pregnancies in hypertension, in Lindheiner M.D., Katz A.L., Zuspan F.R. (eds.): *Hypertension in Pregnancy*. New York, John Wiley & Sons, 1976, p. 329.
482. Still J.G., Greiss F.C. Jr.: The effect of prostaglandin and other vasoactive substances on uterine blood flow and myometrial activity. *Am. J. Obstet. Gynecol.* 130:1–8, 1978.
483. Seino M., Carretero O.A., Albertin R., et al.: Kinins in regulation of uteroplacental blood flow in the pregnant rabbit. *Am. J. Physiol.* 242:142–147, 1982.
484. Bonnar J., Redman C.W.G., Denson K.W.: The role of coagulation and fibrinolysis in preeclampsia, in Lindheimer M.D., Katz A.I., Zuspan F.P.

(eds.): *Hypertension in Pregnancy.* New York, John Wiley & Sons, 1976. pp. 85–94.

485. Ylikorkala O., Viinikka L.: Thromboxane A_2 in pregnancy and puerperium. *Br. Med. J.* 281:1601–1602, 1980.

486. Lewis P.J., Boylan P., Friedman L.A., et al.: Prostacyclin in pregnancy. *Br. Med. J.* 280:1581–1582, 1980.

487. Redman C.W.G., Denson K.W., Beilin L.J., et al.: Factor-VIII consumption in pre-eclampsia. *Lancet* 2:1249–1252, 1977.

488. Weenink G.H., Treffers P.E., Vign P., et al.: Plasma antithrombin II levels in pre-eclampsia. *Clin. Exp. Hypertens.* 2:145–162, 1983.

489. Whigham K.A., Howie P.W., Drummond A.H., et al.: Abnormal platelet function in pre-eclampsia, in Bonnar J., MacGillivray I., Symonds E.M. (eds.): *Pregnancy Hypertension.* Lancaster, England, MTP Press Ltd., 1980, p. 397.

490. Bussolino F., Benedetto C., Massobrio M., et al.: Maternal vascular prostacyclin activity in pre-eclampsia. (letter), *Lancet* 2 (8196):702, 1980.

491. Carreras L.O., Defryn G., Van Houtte E., et al.: Prostacyclin and preeclampsia. *Lancet* 1:442, 1981.

492. Downing I., Shepherd G.L., Lewis P.J.: Reduced prostacyclin production in preeclampsia. *Lancet* 2:1374, 1980.

493. Remuzzi G., Marchesi D., Mecca G.: Reduction of fetal vascular prostacyclin activity in preeclampsia. *Lancet* 2:310, 1980.

494. Faith G.C., Trump B.F.: The glomerular capillary wall in human kidney disease: acute glomerulonephritis, systemic lupus erythematosus, and pre-eclampsia-eclampsia. *Lab. Invest.* 15:1682–1719, 1966.

495. Morris R.H., Vassalli P., Beller F.K., et al.: Immunofluorescent studies of renal biopsies in the diagnosis of toxemia of pregnancy. *Obstet. Gynecol.* 24:32–46, 1964.

496. Petrucco O.M., Thompson N.M., Lawrence O.R., et al.: Immunofluorescent studies in renal biopsies in pre-eclampsia. *Br. Med. J.* 1:473–476, 1974.

497. McKay D.C., Goildenberg V., Kaunitz M., et al.: Experimental eclampsia. *Arch. Pathol.* 84:557–597, 1967.

498. Kaley G., Demopoulas H., Zweifach B.W.: Occlusive vascular lesions induced by bacterial endotoxin in kidneys of pregnant rats. *Proc. Soc. Exp. Biol. Med.* 109:456–459, 1962.

499. Vassalli P., Morris R.H., McCluskey R.T.: The pathogenic role of fibrin deposition in the glomerular lesions of toxemia of pregnancy. *J. Exp. Med.* 118:467–477, 1963.

500. Pritchard J.A., Cunningham F.G., Mason R.A.: Coagulation changes in eclampsia: Their frequency and pathogenesis. *Am. J. Obstet. Gynecol.* 124:855–864, 1976.

501. Altura B.M., Altura B.T.: Magnesium ions and contraction of vascular smooth muscles: relationship to some vascular diseases. *Fed. Proc.* 40:2672–2679, 1981.

502. Altura B.M., Altura B.T., Carella T.A.: Magnesium deficiency-induced spasms of umbilical vessels: Relation to preeclampsia, hypertension, growth retardation. *Science* 221:376–378, 1983.

503. Seelig M.S.: *Magnesium Deficiency in the Pathogenesis of Disease.* New York, Plenum Publishing Corp., 1980.

504. Altura B.M., Altura B.T., Brewold A.: Magnesium deficiency and hypertension: Correlation between magnesium-deficient diets and microcirculatory changes in situ. *Science* 223:1315–1317, 1984.

505. Altura B.M., Altura B.T.: Magnesium ions and contraction of vascular smooth muscles: relationship to some vascular diseases. *Fed. Proc.* 40:2672–2679, 1981.

506. Flowers C.E. Jr.: Magnesium sulfate in obstetrics. A study of magnesium in plasma urine and muscle. *Am. J. Obstet. Gynecol.* 91:763–776, 1965.

507. Lim P., Jacob E., Dong S., et al.: Values for tissue magnesium as a guide in detecting magnesium deficiency. *J. Clin. Path.* 22:417–421, 1969.

508. Hurley L.S.: Trace metals in mammalian development. *Johns Hopkins Med. J.* 148:1–13, 1981.

509. Charbon G., Hoekstra M.: On the competition between calcium and magnesium. *Acta Pharmacol. Neerl.* 11:141–150, 1962.

510. Stitt F.W., Crawford M.D., Clayton D.G., et al.: Clinical and biochemical indicators of cardiovascular disease among men living in hard and soft water areas. *Lancet* 1:122–126, 1973.

511. Masironi R., Kortyohann S.R., Pierce J.O., et al.: Calcium content in river water, trace element concentrations in toenails and blood pressure in village population in New Guinea. *Sci. Total Environ.* 6:41–53, 1976.

512. McCarron D.A., Morris C.D., Cole C.: Dietary calcium in human hypertension. *Science* 217:267–269, 1982.

513. Kesteloot H., Geboers J.: Calcium and blood pressure. *Lancet* 1:813–815, 1982.

514. McCarron D.A.: Blood pressure and calcium balance in the Wistar-Kyoto rat. *Life Sci.* 30:683–689, 1982.

515. Ayachi S.: Increased dietary calcium lowers blood pressure in the spontaneously hypertensive rat. *Metabolism* 28:1234–1238, 1979.

516. McCarron D.A., Yung N.N., Ugoretz B.A., et al.: Disturbances of calcium metabolism in the spontaneously hypertensive rat. *Hypertension* 3:I-162–I-167, 1981.

517. McCarron D.A.: Calcium, magnesium and phosphorus balance in human and experimental hypertension. *Hypertension* 4:III-27–III-33, 1982.

518. Belizan J.M., Pineda O., Sainz E., et al.: Rise of blood pressure in calcium-deprived pregnant rats. *Am. J. Obstet. Gynecol.* 141:163–169, 1981.

519. McCarron D.A., Morria C.: Oral Ca2 + in mild to moderate hypertension: A randomized, placebo-controlled trial. *Clin. Res.* 32:335A, 1984.

520. Allen L.H.: Calcium bioavailability and absorption: a review. *Am. J. Clin. Nutr.* 35:783–808, 1982.

521. Villar J., Belizan J.M., Fischer P.J.: Epidemiologic observations on the relationship between calcium intake and eclampsia. *Int. J. Gynaecol. Obstet.* 21(4):271–278, 1983.

522. Kuriyama H., Ito Y., Suzuki H., et al.: Factors modifying contraction-relaxation cycle in vascular smooth muscles. *Am. J. Physiol.* 243:H641–662, 1982.

523. Christensson T., Hellstrom K., Wengle B.: Clinical and laboratory findings in subjects with hypercalcemia. *Acta Med. Scand.* 200:355–360, 1976.

524. Weidmann P., Massay S.G., Coburn W.J., et al.; Blood pressure effects of acute hypercalcemia: Studies in patients with chronic renal failure. *Ann. Int. Med.* 76:7412–745, 1972.

525. Lueck J., Brewer J., Aladjem S., et al.: Observation of an organism found in patients with gestational trophoblastic disease and in patients with toxemia of pregnancy. *Am. J. Obstet. Gynecol.* 145:15–26, 1983.

526. Aladjem S., Leukck J., Brewer J.: Experimental induction of a toxemia-like syndrome in the pregnant beagle. *Am. J. Obstet. Gynecol.* 145:27–38, 1983.

527. Gau G., Bhundia J., Napher K., et al.: The worm that wasn't. *Lancet* 1:1160–1161, 1983.

528. Richards F.O., Grimes D.A., Wilson M.: The question of a helminthic cause of preeclampsia. *J.A.M.A.* 250:2970–2972, 1983.

529. Beer A.E.: Possible immunologic basis of preeclampsia/eclampsia. *Semin. Perinatol.* 2:39–59, 1978.

530. Adelsberg B.R.: The complement system in pregnancy. *Am. J. Reprod. Immunol.* 4:38–44, 1983.

531. Sinha D., Wells M., Faulk W.P.: Immunologic studies of human placentae: Complement components in preeclamptic chorionic villi. *Clin. Exp. Immunol.* 56(1):175–184, 1984.

532. Anderson J.M.: The effects of transplacental cell (antigen) traffic. *J. Reprod. Fertil.* 31:161–173, 1982.

533. O'Sullivan M.J., McIntyre J.A., Prior M., et al.: Identification of human trophoblast membrane antigens in maternal blood during pregnancy. *Clin. Exp. Immunol.* 48:279–287, 1982.

534. Masson P.L., Deline M., Cambiaso C.L.: Circulating immune complexes in normal human pregnancy. *Nature* 266:542–543, 1977.

535. Stirrat G.M., Redman C.W.G., Levinsky R.J.: Circulating immune complexes in pre-eclampsia. *Br. Med. J.* 1:1450–1451, 1978.

536. D'Amelio R., Bilotta P., Psachi A., et al.: Circulating immune complexes in normal pregnant women and in some conditions complicating pregnancy. *Clin. Exp. Immunol.* 37:33–37, 1979.

537. Persitz, E., Oksenberg J., Amar A., et al.: Histocompatibility antigens, mixed lymphocyte reactivity and severe preeclampsia in Israel. *Gynecol. Obstet. Invest.* 16:283–291, 1983.

538. Medcalf R.L., Kuhn R.J., Iwanov V., et al.: Vasoactivity generated from platelets by immune complexes in pre-eclampsia. *Clin. Exp. Pharmacol. Physiol.* 10:369–373, 1983.

539. Medcalf R.L., Kuhn R.J., Mathews J.D., et al.; Immune complexes and vasoactivity generated from platelets in pre-eclampsia. *Clin. Exp. Hypertens.* 4:511–529, 1982.

540. Vázquez-Escobosa C., Pérez-Medina R., Gómez-Estrada H.: Circulating immune complexes in hypertensive disease of pregnancy. *Obstet. Gynecol.* 62:45–48, 1983.

541. Kuramoto M., Okamura K., Hamazaki Y., et al.: The role of circulating immune-complex in pregnancy. *Tohoku J. Exp. Med.* 138:7–15, 1982.

542. Schena F.P., Manno C., Selvaggi L.: Behaviour of immune complexes and the complement system in normal pregnancy and pre-eclampsia. *J. Clin. Lab. Immunol.* 7:21–26, 1982.

543. Rote N.S., Caudle M.R.; Circulating immune complexes in pregnancy, preeclampsia, and autoimmune diseases: evaluation of Raji cell enzyme-linked immunosorbent assay and polyethylene glycol precipitation methods. *Am. J. Obstet. Gynecol.* 147:267–273, 1983.

544. Knox G.E., Stagno S., Volanakis J.E., et al.: A search for antigen-antibody

complexes in pre-eclampsia: Further evidence against immunologic pathogenesis. *Am. J. Obstet. Gynecol.* 132:87–89, 1978.

545. Pudifin D.J., Moodley J., Duursema J.: Pre-eclamptic toxemia is not associated with elevated levels of circulating immune complexes. (letter), *S. Afr. Med. J.* 63:304–305, 1983.

546. Alanen A., Lassila O.: Cell-mediated immunity in normal pregnancy and pre-eclampsia. *J. Reprod. Immunol.* 4:349–354, 1982.

547. Alanen A., Lassila O.: Deficient natural killer cell function in preeclampsia. *Obstet. Gynecol.* 60:631–634, 1982.

548. Moore M.P., Carter N.P., Redman C.W.: Lymphocyte subsets in normal and pre-eclamptic pregnancies. *Br. J. Obstet. Gynaecol.* 90:326–331, 1982.

549. Gusdon J.P. Jr., Heise E.R., Quinn K.J., et al.: Lymphocyte subpopulations in normal and preeclampsia pregnancies. *Am. J. Reprod. Immunol.* 5:28–31, 1984.

550. Taufield P.A., Sutheranthiran M., Alex, K.: Maternal-fetal immunity: presence of specific cellular hyporesponsiveness and humoral suppressor activity in normal pregnancy and their absence in preeclampsia. *Clin. Exp. Hypertens.* 2:123–131, 1983.

551. Sargent I.L., Redman C.W., Stirrat G.M.: Maternal cell-mediated immunity (CMI) to fetal (paternal) HLA was studied in both normal and preeclamptic pregnancy. *Clin. Exp. Immunol.* 50:601–609, 1982.

552. Sridama V., Yang S.L., Moawad A., et al.: T-cell subsets in patients with preeclampsia. *Am. J. Obstet. Gynecol.* 147:4566–569, 1983.

553. Pietarinen I., Kivinen S., Ylostalo P., et al.: Smooth muscle antibodies in preeclampsia of pregnancy. *Gynecol. Obstet. Invest.* 13:142–149, 1982.

554. Riva-Rocci S.: Un nuovo sfigmonometro. *Gazz. Med. Torino* 47:981–1001, 1896.

555. Schottstaedt M.F., Sokolow M.: The natural history and course of hypertension with papilledema (malignant hypertension). *Am. Heart J.* 45:331–362, 1953.

556. McMichael J., Murphy E.A.: Methonium treatment of severe and malignant hypertension. *J. Chronic Dis.* 1:527–535, 1955.

557. Kincaid-Smith P., McMichael J., Murphy E.A.: The clinical course and pathology of hypertension with papilloedema (malignant hypertension). *Q. J. Med.* 27:117–153, 1958.

558. Perry H.M. Jr., Schroeder H.A., Catanzara F.J., et al.: Studies on the control of hypertension. VIII. Mortality, morbidity, and remission during twelve years of intensive therapy. *Circulation* 33:958–972, 1966.

559. Sokolow M., Perloff D.: Five-year survival of consecutive patients with malignant hypertension treated with antihypertensive agents. *Am. J. Cardiol.* 6:858–863, 1960.

560. Woods J.W., Blythe W.B.: Management of malignant hypertension complicated by renal insufficiency. *New Engl. J. Med.* 277:57–61. 1967.

561. Hodge J.V., Smirk F.H.: The effect of drug treatment of hypertension on the distribution of deaths from various causes. A study of 173 deaths among hypertensive patients in the years 1959 to 1964 inclusive. *Am. Heart J.* 73:441–452, 1967.

562. Build and Blood Pressure Study, *Chicago Society of Actuaries,* vol. 2. 1959.

563. Blood Pressure Study 1979. Society of Actuaries and Association of Life Insurance Medical Directors of America, 1979.

564. Kannel W.B., Castelli W.P., McNamara P.M., et al.: The Framingham Study: Some factors affecting morbidity and mortality in hypertension. *Milbank Mem. Fund Q.* 47(3):116–142, Part 2, 1969.

565. Kannel W.B., Schwartz M.J., McNamara P.M.: Blood pressure and risk of coronary heart disease. The Framingham study. *Dis. Chest* 56:43–52, 1969.

566. United States National Center for Health Statistics. Vital and Health Statistics. *Heart Disease in Adults: United States, 1960–1962* (PHS Publication No. 1000, Series 11, No. 6). Washington, D.C., Government Printing Office, 1964.

567. Stamler J., Kjelsberg M., Hall Y.: Epidemiologic studies on cardiovascular-renal disease. I. Analysis of mortality by age-race-sex-occupation. *J. Chronic Dis.* 12:440–455, 1960.

568. Byrom F.B.: Pathogenesis of hypertensive encephalopathy and relation to malignant phase of hypertension: experimental evidence from hypertensive rat. *Lancet* 2:201–211, 1954.

569. Sako Y.: Effect of turbulent blood flow and hypertension on experimental atherosclerosis. *J.A.M.A.* 179:36–40, 1962.

570. Heath D., Wood E.H., Dushane J.W., et al.; The relation of age and blood pressure to atheroma in the pulmonary arteries and thoracic aorta in congenital heart disease. *Lab. Invest.* 9:259–272, 1960.

571. Brust A.A., Ferris E.B.: Diagnostic approach to hypertension due to unilateral kidney disease. *Ann. Intern. Med.* 47:1049–1066, 1957.

572. Gaunt R., Antonchak N., Miller G.J., et al.: Effect of reserpine (Serpasil) and hydralazine (Apresoline) on experimental steroid hypertension. *Amer. J. Physiol.* 182:63–68, 1955.

573. Perry H.M. Jr., Schroeder H.A.: The effect of treatment on mortality rates in severe hypertension. A comparison of medical and surgical regimens. *Arch. Intern. Med.* 102:418–428, 1958.

574. Dustan H.P., Schneckloth R.E., Corcoran A.C., et al.: The effectiveness of long-term treatment of malignant hypertension. *Circulation* 18:644–651, 1958.

575. Hamilton M., Thompson E.N., Wisniewski T.K.M.: The role of blood pressure control in preventing complications of hypertension. *Lancet* 1:235–238, 1964.

576. Wolff F.W., Lindeman R.D.: Effects of treatment on hypertension: results of a controlled study. *J. Chronic Dis.* 19:227–240, 1966.

577. Veterans Administration Cooperative Study Group on Antihypertensive Agents. Effect of treatment on morbidity: Results in patients with diastolic blood pressure averaging 115 through 129 mm Hg. *J.A.M.A.* 213:1143–1152, 1970.

578. Veterans Administration Cooperative Study Group on Antihypertensive Agents. Effect of treatment on morbidity: results in patients with diastolic blood pressure averaging 90 through 114 mmHg. *J.A.M.A.* 213:1143–1152, 1970.

579. Veterans Administration Cooperative Study Group on Antihypertensive Agents. Effects of treatment on morbidity in hypertension: III. Influence of age, diastolic pressure, and prior cardiovascular disease, further analysis of side effects. *Circulation* 45:991–1004, 1972.

580. Hypertension Detection and Follow-Up Program Cooperative Group: Four-Year Findings of the Hypertension Detection and Follow-up Pro-

gram. 1. Reduction in mortality of persons with high blood pressure, including mild hypertension. *J.A.M.A.* 242:2562–2571, 1979.

581. The Australian Therapeutic Trial in Mild Hypertension. Report by the Management Committee. *Lancet* 1:1261–1267, June 14, 1980.

582. Friedman E.A., Neff R.K.: Hypertension and hypotension in pregnancy, correlation with fetal outcome. *J.A.M.A.* 239:2249–2251, 1978.

583. Page E.W., Christianson R.: The impact of mean arterial pressure in the middle trimester upon the outcome of pregnancy. *Am. J. Obstet. Gynecol.* 125:740–746, 1976.

584. Browne J.C.M., Veall N.: The maternal placental blood flow in normotensive and hypertensive women. *J. Obstet. Gynaecol. Br. Commonw.* 60:141–147, 1953.

585. Sibai B.M., Abdella T.N., Anderson G.D.: Pregnancy outcome in 211 patients with mild chronic hypertension. *Obstet. Gynecol.* 61:571–576, 1983.

586. Feitelson P.J., Lindheimer M.D.: Management of hypertensive gravidas. *J. Reprod. Med.* 8:111–116, 1972.

587. Dunlop J.C.H.: Chronic hypertension and perinatal mortality. *Proc. R. Soc. Lond.* 59:838–841, 1966.

588. Robertson E.G.: The natural history of oedema during pregnancy. *J. Obstet. Gynaecol. Br. Commonw.* 78:520–529, 1971.

589. Chesley L.C.: Eclampsia: The remote prognosis. *Seminars in Perinatology* 2:99–111, 1978.

590. Bryans C.I. Jr.: The remote prognosis of toxemia of pregnancy. *Clin. Obstet. Gynecol.* 9:973–990, 1966.

591. Chesley L.C., Annitto J.E., Cosgrove R.A.: The remote prognosis of eclamptic women: sixth periodic report. *Am. J. Obstet. Gynecol.* 124:446–459, 1976.

592. Hamilton M., Pickering G.W., Roberts J.A.F., et al.: The etiology of essential hypertension. I. The arterial blood pressure in the general population. *Clin. Sci.* 13:11–35, 1954.

593. Svensson A., Andersch B., Hansson L.: A clinical follow-up study of 260 women with hypertension in pregnancy. *Clin. Exp. Hypertens.* 2:95–102, 1983.

594. Sullivan J.M.: Management of essential hypertension during pregnancy. *Clin. Cardiol.* 2:368–374, 1979.

595. Ueland K., Hansen J.M.: Maternal cardiovascular dynamics. III. Labor and delivery under local and caudal analgesia. *Amer. J. Obstet. Gynecol.* 103:8–18, 1969.

596. Chamberlain, G.V.P., Lewis P.J., Swiet M.D., et al.: How obstetricians manage hypertension in pregnancy. *Br. Med. J.* 1:626–629, 1978.

597. Curet L.B., Olson R.W.: Evaluation of a program of bed rest in the treatment of chronic hypertension in pregnancy. *Obstet. Gynecol.* 53:336–340, 1979.

598. Mathews D.D.: A randomized controlled trial of bed rest and sedation or normal activity and non-sedation in the management of non-albuminuric hypertension in late pregnancy. *Br. J. Obstet. Gynaecol.* 84:108–114, 1977.

599. Pritchard J.A.: Management of severe preeclampsia and eclampsia. *Semin. Perinatol.* 2:83–97, 1978.

600. Cunningham F.G., Pritchard J.A.: How should hypertension during preg-

nancy be managed? Experience at Parkland Memorial Hospital. *Med. Clin. North Am.* 68:505–526, 1984.

601. Lindheimer M.D., Katz A.L.: Sodium and diuretics in pregnancy. *N. Engl. J. Med.* 288:891–894, 1973.

602. Pritchard J.A.: Changes in blood volume during pregnancy and delivery. *Anesthesiology* 26:393–399, 1965.

603. Hytten F.E., Paintin D.B.: Increases in plasma volume during normal pregnancy. *J. Obstet. Gynaecol. Br. Commonw.* 70:402–407, 1963.

604. Gray M.J., Munro A.B., Sims E.A.H., et al.: Regulation of sodium and total body water metabolism in pregnancy. *Am. J. Obstet. Gynecol.* 89:760–765, 1964.

605. Sims E.A.H., Krantz K.E.: Serial studies of renal function during pregnancy and the puerperium in normal women. *J. Clin. Invest.* 37:1764–1774, 1958.

606. Lin T.J., Lin S.C., Erlenmeyer F., et al.: Progesterone production rates during the third trimester of pregnancy in normal women, diabetic women and women with abnormal glucose tolerance. *J. Clin. Endocrinol. Metab.* 34:287–297, 1972.

607. Landau R.L., Lugibihl K.: Inhibition of the sodium retaining influence of aldosterone by progesterone. *J. Clin. Endocrinol. Metab.* 18:1237–1245, 1958.

608. Crane M.G., Harris J.J.: Plasma renin activity and aldosterone excretion rate in normal subjects: 1. Effect of ethinyl estradiol and medroxyprogesterone acetate. *J. Clin. Endocrinol. Metab.* 29:550–557, 1969.

609. Watanabe M., Meeker M.L., Gray M.J., et al.: Secretion of aldosterone in normal pregnancy. *J. Clin. Invest.* 42:1619–1631, 1963.

610. Boonshaft B., O'Connell J.M.B., Hayes J.M., et al.: Serum renin activity during normal pregnancy: Effect of alterations of posture and sodium intake. *J. Clin. Endocrinol. Metab.* 28:1641–1644, 1968.

611. Ehrlich E.N., Lugibihl K., Taylor C., et al.: Reciprocal variations in urinary cortisol and aldosterone in response to the sodium-depleting influence of hydrochlorothiazide and ethacrynic acid in humans. *J. Clin. Endocrinol. Metab.* 27:836–842, 1967.

612. Weinberger M.H., Kraner N.J., Grim C.E., et al.: The effect of posture and saline loading on plasma renin activity and aldosterone concentration in pregnant, non-pregnant and estrogen treated women. *J. Clin. Endocrinol. Metab.* 44:69–77, 1977.

613. Biglieri E.G., Slaton P.E., Kronfield S.J., et al.: Diagnosis of an aldosterone-producing adenoma in primary aldosteronism. An evaluative maneuver. *J.A.M.A.* 201:510–514, 1967.

614. Ehrlich E.N.: Heparinoid-induced inhibition of aldosterone secretion in normal pregnant women. The rate of augmented aldosterone secretion in sodium conservation during normal pregnancy. *Am. J. Obstet. Gynecol.* 109:963–970, 1971.

615. Chesley L.C.: Plasma and red cell volumes during pregnancy. *Am. J. Obstet. Gynecol.* 112:440–450, 1972.

616. Blekta M., Hlavaty V., Trinkova M., et al.: Volume of whole blood and absolute amount of serum proteins in the early stage of late toxemia of pregnancy. *Am. J. Obstet. Gynecol.* 106:10–13, 1970.

617. Lang G.D., Lowe G.D., Walker J.J., et al.: Blood rheology in preeclampsia and intrauterine growth retardation: effects of blood pressure reduction with labetalol. *Br. J. Obstet. Gynaecol.* 91:438–443, 1984.

618. Arias F.: Expansion of intravascular volume and fetal outcome in patients with chronic hypertension and pregnancy. *Am. J. Obstet. Gynecol.* 123:610–616, 1975.

619. Soffronoff E.C., Kaufmann B.M., Connaughton J.F.: Intravascular volume determinations and fetal outcome in hypertensive diseases of pregnancy. *Am. J. Obstet. Gynecol.* 127:4–9, 1977.

620. Gallery E.D.M., Hunyor S.N., Gyory A.Z.: Plasma volume contraction. A significant factor in both pregnancy-associated hypertension (preeclampsia) and chronic hypertension in pregnancy. *Q. J. Med.* 192:593–602, 1979.

621. Benedetti T.J., Carlson R.W.: Studies of colloid osmotic pressure in pregnancy-induced hypertension. *Am. J. Obstet. Gynecol.* 135(3):308–311, 1979.

621a. Goddlin R., Kurpershoek C., Haesslein H.: Colloid osmotic pressure changes during hypertensive pregnancy. *Clin. Exp. Hypertens.* 1:49–56, 1982.

622. Robinson M.: Salt in pregnancy. *Lancet* 1:178–181, 1958.

623. Zuspan F.P., Bell J.D.: Variable salt loading during pregnancy with preeclampsia. *Obstet. Gynecol.* 18:530–534, 1961.

624. Mengert W.F., Tacchi D.A.: Pregnancy toxemia and sodium chloride. *Am. J. Obstet. Gynecol.* 81:601–605, 1961.

625. Bower D.: The influence of dietary salt intake on preeclampsia. *J. Obstet. Gynaecol. Br. Commonw.* 71:123–125, 1964.

626. Foote R.G., Ludbrook A.P.R.: The use of liberal salt diet in preeclamptic toxaemia and essential hypertension with pregnancy. *N. Z. Med. J.* 77:242–245, 1973.

627. Wilson I.M., Freis E.D.: Relationship between plasma and extracellular fluid volume depletion and the antihypertensive effect of chlorothiazide. *Circulation* 20:1028–1036, 1959.

628. Dustan H.P., Cumming G.R., Corcoran A.C., et al.: A mechanism of chlorothiazide-enhanced effectiveness of antihypertensive ganglioplegic drugs. *Circulation* 19:360–365, 1959.

629. Dollery C.T., Harington M., Kaufman G.: The mode of action of chlorothiazide in hypertension: with special reference to potentiation of ganglioblocking agents. *Lancet* 1:1215–1218, 1959.

630. Lauwers P., Conway J.: Effect of long-term treatment with chlorothiazide on body fluids, serum electrolytes, and exchangeable sodium in hypertensive patients. *J. Lab. Clin. Med.* 56:401–408, 1960.

631. Tobian L.: Why do thiazide diuretics lower blood pressure in essential hypertension? *Ann. Rev. Pharmacol.* 7:399–408, 1967.

632. Daniel E.E.: On the mechanism of antihypertensive action of hydrochlorothiazide in rats. *Circ. Res.* 11:941–954, 1962.

633. Tobian L., Janecek J., Foker J., et al.: Effect of chlorothiazide on renal juxtaglomerular cells and tissue electrolytes. *Am. J. Physiol.* 202:905–908, 1962.

634. Weller J.M., Haight A.S.: Effect of chlorothiazide on blood pressure and electrolytes of normotensive and hypertensive rats. *Proc. Soc. Exp. Biol. Med.* 112:820–825, 1963.

635. Tarazi R.C., Dustan H.P., Frohlich E.D.: Long-term thiazide therapy in essential hypertension. Evidence for persistent alteration in plasma volume and renin activity. *Circulation* 41:709–717, 1970.

636. Finnerty F.A. Jr., Bucklholz J.H., Tuckman J.:.Evaluation of chlorothiazide (Diuril) in the toxemia of pregnancy. *J.A.M.A.* 166:141–144, 1958.

637. Salerno L.J., Stone M.L., Ditchik P.: A clinical evaluation of chlorothiazide in prevention and treatment of toxemia of pregnancy. *Obstet. Gynecol.* 14:188–192, 1959.

638. MacGillivray I., Hytten F.E., Taggart N., et al.: The effect of a sodium diuretic on total exchangeable sodium and total body water in preeclamptic toxaemia. *J. Obstet. Gynaecol. Br. Commonw.* 69:458–462, 1962.

639. Finnerty F.A. Jr., Bepko F.J. Jr.: Lowering of the perinatal mortality and the prematurity rate. The value of prophylactic thiazides in juvenile pregnancy. *J.A.M.A.* 195:429–432, 1966.

640. Kraus G.W., Marchese J.R., Yen S.S.C.: Prophylactic use of hydrochlorothiazide in pregnancy. *J.A.M.A.* 198:1150–1154, 1966.

641. Brewer Th.H.: Administration serum albumin in severe acute toxemia of pregnancy. *J. Obstet. Gynaecol. Br. Commonw.* 70:1001–1004, 1963.

642. Obolensky W., Wenzel K.: Plasma expanders in the treatment of gestosis, II. *Internatl. Symp. über EPH Gestose*, Oct. 1972 in Aarau, Switzerland.

643. Schwarz R., Retzhe U.: Die kardio-vaskulare Werkung von niedermolskularem Dextran bei hypertensiven Spatschwangeren. *Zentra lbl. Gynaekol.* 90:557–586, 1968.

644. Vara P.: Observations in the use of 10% salt-free macrodex in toxemia of late pregnancy. *Acta Obstet. Gynecol. Scand.* 30(Suppl. 6):1–32, 1950.

645. Cloeren S.E., Lippert T.H., Hinselmann H.: Hypovolemia in toxemia of pregnancy: Plasma expander therapy with surveillance of central venous pressure. *Arch. Gynec.* 215:123–132, 1973.

646. Goodlin R.C., Cotton D.P., Haesslein H.C.: Severe edema-proteinuria gestosis. *Am. J. Obstet. Gynecol.* 132:595–598, 1978.

647. Maclean A.B., Doig J.R., Alckin D.R.: Hypovolemia, pre-eclampsia and diuretics. *Br. J. Obstet. Gynecol.* 85:597–601, 1978.

648. Jouppila P., Jouppila R., Koivula A.: Albumin infusion does not alter the intervillous blood flow in severe pre-eclampsia. *Acta Obstet. Gynecol. Scand.* 62:345–348, 1983.

649. Goodlin R.C., Dobry C.A., Anderson J.C., et al.: Clinical signs of normal plasma volume expansion during pregnancy. *Am. J. Obstet. Gynecol.* 145:1001–1009, 1983.

650. Redman C.W.G.: Maternal plasma volume and disorders of pregnancy. *Br. Med. J.* 288:955–956, 1984.

651. Kincaid-Smith P., Bullen M., Mills J.: Prolonged use of methyldopa in severe hypertension in pregnancy. *Br. Med. J.* 1:274–276, 1966.

652. Leather H.M., Hymphreys D.M., Baker P., et al.: A controlled trial of hypertensive agents in hypertension in pregnancy. *Lancet* 2:488–490, 1968.

653. Redman C.W.G., Beilin L.J., Bonnar J., et al.: Fetal outcome in trial of antihypertensive treatment in pregnancy. *Lancet* 2:753–756, 1976.

654. Ounsted M.K., Moar V.A., Good F.J., et al.: Hypertension during pregnancy with and without specific treatment; the development of the children at the age of four years. *Br. J. Obstet. Gynaecol.* 87:19–24, 1980.

655. Eliahou H.E., Silverberg D.S., Reisen E., et al.: Propranolol for the treatment of hypertension in pregnancy. *Br. J. Obstet. Gynaecol.* 85:431–436, 1978.

656. Tcherdakoff P.H., Colliard M., Berrard E., et al.: Propranolol in hypertension during pregnancy. *Br. Med. J.* 2:670, 1978.

657. Lieberman B.A., Stirrat G.M., Cohen S.L., et al.: The possible adverse effect of propranolol on the fetus in pregnancies complicated by severe hypertension. *Br. J. Obstet. Gynaecol.* 85:678–683, 1978.

658. Pruyn S.C., Phelan J.P., Buchanan G.C.: Long-term propranolol therapy in pregnancy: maternal and fetal outcome. *Am. J. Obstet. Gynecol.* 135:485–489, 1979.

659. O'Hare M.F., Russell C.J., Leahey W.J., et al.: Sotalol in the management of hypertension complicating pregnancy. *Br. J. Clin. Pharmacol.* 8:390P–391P, 1979.

660. Sandstrom B.: Antihypertensive treatment with the adrenergic beta-receptor blocker metoprolol during pregnancy. *Gynecol. Invest.* 9:195–204, 1978.

661. Michael C.A.: Use of labetalol in the treatment of severe hypertension during pregnancy. *Br. J. Clin. Pharmacol.* 8(Suppl 2):211S–215S, 1979.

662. Lunell N.O., Nylund L., Lewander R., et al.: Acute effect of an antihypertensive drug, labetalol, on uteroplacental blood flow. *Br. J. Obstet. Gynaecol.* 89:640–644, 1982.

663. Lamming G.D., Symonds E.B.: Use of labetalol and methyldopa in pregnancy-induced hypertension. *Br. J. Clin. Pharmacol.* 8(Suppl 2):217S–222S, 1979.

664. Gallery E.D., Saunders D.M., Hunyor S.N., et al.: Randomised comparison of methyldopa and oxprenolol for treatment of hypertension in pregnancy. *Br. Med. J.* 1(6178):1591–1594, 1979.

665. Rubin P.C., Clark D.M., Sumner D.J., et al.: Placebo-controlled trial of atenolol in treatment of pregnancy-associated hypertension. *Lancet* 1:431–434, 1983.

666. Lund-Johansen P.: Hemodynamic consequences of long-term beta-blocker therapy: A 5-year follow-up study of atenolol. *J. Cardiovasc. Pharmacol.* 1:487–495, 1979.

667. Johnson T., Clayton C.G.: Diffusion of radioactive sodium in normotensive and preeclamptic pregnancies. *Br. Med. J.* 1:312–314, 1957.

668. Gant N.F., Madden J.D., Siiteri P.K., et al.: The metabolic clearance rate of dehydroisoandrosterone sulfate. IV. Acute effects of induced hypertension, and natriuresis in normal and hypertensive pregnancies. *Am. J. Obstet. Gynecol.* 124:143–148, 1976.

669. Lunell N.O., Lewander R., Nylund L., et al.: Acute effect of dihydralazine on uteroplacental blood flow in hypertension during pregnancy. *Gynecol. Obstet. Invest.* 16:274–282, 1983.

670. Vink G.J., Moodley J., Philpott R.H.: Effect of dihydralazine on the fetus in the treatment of maternal hypertension. *Obstet. Gynecol.* 55:519–522, 1980.

671. Bott-Kanner G., Schweitzer A., Reisner S.H., et al.: Propranolol and hydralazine in the management of essential hypertension in pregnancy. *Br. J. Obstet. Gynaecol.* 87:110–114, 1980.

672. Sullivan J.M., Palmer E.T., Schoeneberger A.A., et al.: SQ 20,881: Effect

on eclamptic-preeclamptic women with postpartum hypertension. *Am. J. Obstet. Gynecol.* 131:707–715, 1978.

673. Pipkin F.B., Turner S.R., Symonds E.M.: Possible risk with captopril in pregnancy; some animal data. (Letter), *Lancet* 1:1256, 1980.

674. Ferris T.F., Weir E.K.: The effect of captopril on uterine blood flow and PGE synthesis in the pregnant rabbit. *J. Clin. Invest.* 71:809–885, 1983.

675. Turner G., Collins E.: Fetal effects of regular salicylate ingestion in pregnancy. *Lancet* 2:338–339, 1975.

676. Shapiro S., Monson R.R., Kaufman D.W., et al.: Perinatal mortality and birth weight in relation in aspirin taken during pregnancy. *Lancet* 1:1375–1376, 1976.

677. Singh B.N., Heght H.S., Nademaneg K., et al.: Electrophysiological and hemodynamic actions of slow channel blocking compounds. *Progr. Cardiovasc. Dis.* 25:103–132, 1982.

678. Zaret G.M.: Possible treatment of pre-eclampsia with calcium channel blocking agents. *Med. Hypotheses* 12:303–319, 1983.

679. Sammour M.B., El-makhzangy M.N., Fawzy M.M., et al.; Progesterone therapy in pregnancy induced hypertension. Therapeutic value and hormonal profile. *Clin. Exp. Hypertens.* 1:455–478, 1982.

680. Sullivan J.M.: Physiologic and biochemical profile of hypertension for rational clinical management, in Stollerman G.H. (ed.): *Advances in Internal Medicine,* vol. 23. Chicago, Year Book Medical Publishers, Inc., 1978.

681. Laragh J.H.: Vasoconstriction-volume analysis for understanding and testing hypertension: The use of renin and aldosterone profiles. *Am. J. Med.* 55:261–274, 1977.

682. Lim Y.L., Walters W.A.: Haemodynamics of mild hypertension in pregnancy. *Br. J. Obstet. Gynaecol.* 86:198–204, 1979.

683. Lees M.M.: Central circulatory responses in normotensive and hypertensive pregnancy. *Postgrad. Med. J.* 55:311–314, 1979.

684. Werkö L.: Studies in the problems of circulation in pregnancy, in Hammond J., Browne F.J., Wolsterholme G.E.W. (eds.): *Toxaemias of Pregnancy.* Ciba Foundation Symposium, London, Churchill-Livingstone, 1950, p. 155.

685. Gant N.F., Daley G.L., Chand S., et al.: A study of angiotensin II pressor response throughout primigravid pregnancy. *J. Clin. Invest.* 52:2682–2689, 1973.

686. Sullivan J.M.: Blood pressure elevation in pregnancy. *Prog. Cardiovasc. Dis.* 16:375–393, 1974.

687. Feinberg L.E.: Hypertension and Preeclampsia, in Abrams R.S., Wexler P. (eds.): *Medical Care of the Pregnant Patient.* Boston, Toronto, Little, Brown & Co., 1983, pp. 161–182.

688. Gant N.F. Jr., Worley R.J.: *Hypertension in Pregnancy, Concepts and Management.* New York, Appleton-Century-Crofts, 1980.

689. Schewitz L.J., Friedman I.A., Pollack V.E.: Bleeding after renal biopsy in pregnancy. *Obstet. Gynecol.* 26:295–304, 1965.

690. Chesley L.C.: Hypertensive disorders in pregnancy, in Hellman L.M., Pritchard J.A. (eds.): *William's Obstetrics.* New York, Appleton-Century-Crofts, 1971, p. 685.

691. Gilstrap L.C., Cunningham F.G., Whalle P.J.: Management of pregnancy-

induced hypertension in the nulliparous patient remote from term. *Semin. Perinatol.* 2:73–81, 1978.

692. Gallery E.D.M., Nunyor S.N., Gyory A.Z.: Plasma volume contraction: A significant factor in both pregnancy-associated hypertension (pre-eclampsia) and chronic hypertension in pregnancy. *Q. J. Med.* 48:593–602, 1979.

693. Assali N.S.: Hemodynamic effects of hypotensive drugs used in obstetrics. *Obstet. Gynecol. Survey* 9:776–794, 1954.

694. Reid D.E.: Hypertensive (toxemic) pregnancy, in Reid D.E., Ryan K.J., Benirschke K. (eds.): *Principals and Management of Human Reproduction.* Philadelphia, W.B. Saunders Co., 1972.

695. Landesman R., Halpern M., Krapp R.C.: Renal artery lesions associated with the toxemias of pregnancy. *Obstet. Gynecol.* 18:645–652, 1961.

696. Dill L.U., Erickson C.C.: Eclampsia-like syndrome occurring in pregnant dogs and rabbits following renal artery constriction. *Proc. Soc. Exp. Biol. Med.* 39:362–365, 1938.

697. Corbit J.D. Jr.: The effect of pregnancy upon experimental hypertension in the rabbit. *Am. J. Med. Sci.* 201:876–884, 1941.

698. Page E.W., Patton H.S., Ogden E.: The effect of pregnancy on experimental hypertension with observations on the effects of deciduomas. *Am. J. Obstet. Gynecol.* 41:53–60, 1941.

699. Schewitz L.J.: Hypertension and renal disease in pregnancy. *Med. Clin. North Am.* 55:47–69, 1971.

700. Fox L.P., Grandi J., Johnson M.J.; Pheochromocytoma associated with pregnancy. *Am. J. Obstet. Gynecol.* 104:288–295, 1966.

701. Hendee A.E., Martin R.D., Waters W.C. III: Hypertension in pregnancy: toxemia or pheochromocytoma? *Am. J. Obstet. Gynecol.* 105:64–72, 1969.

702. Biglieri E.G., Slaton P.E. Jr.: Pregnancy and primary aldosteronism, *J. Clin. Endocrinol.* 27:1628–1632, 1967.

703. Boucher B.J., Mason A.S.: Conn's syndrome with associated pregnancy. *Proc. R. Soc. Med.* 58:575–576, 1965.

704. Hunt A.B., McConahey W.M.: Pregnancy associated with disease of the adrenal glands. *Am. J. Obstet. Gynecol.* 66:970–987, 1953.

705. Shanahan W.R., Romney S.L., Currens J.H.: Coarctation of the aorta and pregnancy. *J.A.M.A.* 167:275–280, 1958.

706. Chemetson C.A.B.: Aortic hypoplasia and its significance in the aetiology of pre-eclamptic toxaemia. *J. Obstet. Gynaecol. Br. Emp.* 67:90–101, 1960.

707. Gordon G., McKay R.T.: Pre-eclampsia associated with hypoplasia of the aorta. *J. Obstet. Gynaecol. Br. Commonw.* 71:785–787, 1964.

708. Chesley L.C., Annitto J.E., Cosgrove R.A.; Long-term follow-up study of eclamptic women. *Am. J. Obstet. Gynecol.* 101:886–898, 1968.

709. Hirsch M.R., Mark M.S.: Pseudotoxemia and erythroblastosis: Report of a case. *Obstet. Gynecol.* 24:47–48, 1964.

710. John A.H., Duncan A.S.: The maternal syndrome associated with hydrops foetalis. *J. Obstet. Gynaecol. Br. Commonw.* 71:61–65, 1964.

711. MacGillivray I., Rose G.A., Rowe B.: Blood pressure survey in pregnancy. *Clin. Sci.* 37:394–407, 1969.

712. Eich R.H., Cuddy R.P., Smulyan H., et al.: Hemodynamics in labile hypertension. A follow-up study. *Circulation* 34:299–307, 1966.

713. Greiss F.C. Jr.: Pressure-flow relationship in the gravid uterine vascular bed. *Am. J. Obstet. Gynecol.* 96:41–47, 1966.

714. Venuto R.C., Cox J.W., Stein J.H., et al.: The effect of changes in perfusion pressure on uteroplacental blood flow in the pregnant rabbit. *J. Clin. Invest.* 57:938–944, 1976.

715. Arias F., Zamora J.: Antihypertensive treatment and pregnancy outcome in patients with mild, chronic hypertension. *Obstet. Gynecol.* 53:489–494, 1979.

716. Horuath T.S., Phippard A., Smart D.H., et al.: High-risk hypertensive pregnancies. Maternal and fetal outcome. *Clin Exp. Hypertens.* 2:21–28, 1982.

717. Department of Health and Social Security. Report on confidential enquiries into maternal deaths in England and Wales 1973–1975, London, HM50, 21–9, 1979.

INDEX

A

Abuse: analgesic, nephropathy of, 55
ACTH, 86
Activity: and hypertension, 127–131
Adenosine, 11
  triphosphate, 43
ADH, 29
  prostaglandins and, 45
ADP, 43
Adrenal disease: hypertension
  secondary to, 162
Adrenergic transmission, 47
α-Adrenergic receptors, 35
β-Adrenergic blockers, 41
β-Adrenergic receptor blockers, 35,
  38
  adverse effects, 141
  in hypertension during pregnancy,
  140–141
Adrenocorticosteroids, 86
Afterload, 12
Albumin infusion
  intervillous blood flow after, 138
  intravenous, 137
Aldosterone
  acting directly on tissues, 38
  in preeclampsia, 87
  -renin-angiotensin (see Renin,
    -angiotensin-aldosterone)
  secretion, 87
Aldosteronism
  primary, 38, 162
  secondary, 162
Alpha-adrenergic receptors, 35
Aminoglutethimide, 41
Amniocentesis: for fetal evaluation,
  152
Amobarbital, 154
Analgesic abuse: nephropathy of, 55

Aneurysm: dissecting, 122
Angiotensin
  -converting enzyme, 36, 61
    blocker, arterial blood pressure
    after, 149
  inhibitors, 143–144
  -renin-aldosterone (see Renin,
    -angiotensin-aldosterone)
  tachyphylaxis, 47
  II, 11
    acting directly on tissues, 38
    generation in hypertensive
    vascular disease, 40
    indomethacin and, 91
    loss of sensitivity to, 47
    during pregnancy, 86
    pressor response to, 80–81
    prostaglandin release and, 55–56
Antibody(ies)
  blocking, and immune response in
    preeclampsia, 97
  maternal, against fetal antigens, 98
  monoclonal, 100
    anti-T-cell, 100
  muscle, smooth, 100
Antidiuretic factors: in preeclampsia,
  88
Antidiuretic hormone, 29
  prostaglandins and, 45
Antigen(s)
  fetal, maternal recognition of, 98
  trophoblast-specific membrane, 98
Antihypertensive agents, 126–127
  adverse effects, 128–130
  precautions during pregnancy, 145,
  146
Antihypertensive management,
  123–146
  general considerations, 123–125
  during pregnancy, 125–146

Antihypertensive medullary lipids
(*see* Lipids, antihypertensive
medullary)
Antihypertensive therapy
goals of, 121–123
during pregnancy, 122
Anti-inflammatory agents:
nonsteroidal, 57, 89
Antithrombin III, 93
Aorta, 9
coarctation, hypertension
secondary to, 162
hypoplasia, 163
Arachidonic acid: metabolism by
prostaglandin synthetase
complex, 46
Arteries
muscular, 9
pressure
diastolic, relationship with
plasma volume, 24
long-term level analysis, 23
renal, stenosis, unilateral, 63
Arterioles
local factors influencing, 10
remote factors influencing, 10
resistance, 9
Aspirin
fetal mortality after, 143–144
inhibiting cyclooxygenase activity,
52
Atenolol, 141
Atherosclerosis: accelerated,
complications related to, 107
ATPase
potassium, 30
sodium-potassium, 83
Atrium, 9
left, stretch receptors of, 29
natriuretic factor, 29, 83
Autonomic nervous system, 9
activity increase, 20
in borderline hypertension, 21
in labile hypertension, 20
in preeclampsia, 82
Autoregulation
of circulation, 9, 11
local, 43
stimulation of, 22

of uterine blood flow, 165
whole-body, 26

B

Baroreceptor reflex, 25
Bartter's syndrome, 57
Bayliss effect, 11, 43
Bed rest, 127
in preeclampsia, 152
Beta-adrenergic blockers, 41
Beta-adrenergic receptor blockers, 35,
38
adverse effects, 141
in hypertension during pregnancy,
140–141
17-Beta-estradiol, 85
Blacks: prevalence of hypertension
in, 1
Blockade
beta-adrenergic receptor, 38
of prostaglandin synthesis, 49
Blocker
angiotensin-converting enzyme,
149
beta-adrenergic, 41
beta-adrenergic receptor, 35
adverse effects of, 141
in hypertension during
pregnancy, 140–141
calcium channel, 42
for hypertension during
pregnancy, 144
of sympathetic nervous system,
139–140
Blood
flow
cerebral, 79
after diazoxide, 167
intervillous, after albumin
infusion, 138
liver, in pregnancy-induced
hypertension, 79
muscle, in pregnancy-induced
hypertension, 79
renal, 44, 49, 61, 82
uterine, 13, 42, 79
uterine, autoregulation of, 165

uterine, effect of varying
  perfusion on, 168
uterine, elevation, and
  prostaglandin E_2, 89
uteroplacental, 74, 165
uteroplacental, after hydralazine,
  142
platelets (see Platelets)
pressure
  control, optimal, 165–168
  after diazoxide, 167
  diurnal variation, 79
  after eclampsia, 118, 119
  elevated (see below)
  high, complications related to,
    106–107
  high, fetal mortality and, 114
  high, risk factors related to,
    106
  primigravidas, 17
  regulation, 43
  regulation, kidney in, 53
  Study of U.S. Society of
    Actuaries, 105
pressure, elevated, 103–111
  consequences of, 103–111
  malignant phase of, 103
  during pregnancy,
    consequences, 113–120
  severely, 103
  treatment, rationale for, 106–111
vessels (see Vessels)
volume, 13–14, 131
  (See also Volume)
  in borderline hypertension,
    21
  changes during pregnancy, 14
  effective, 42
  in preeclampsia, 133
  in pregnancy-induced
    hypertension, 79
Bradycardia: of newborn, 140
Bradykinin, 11, 59
Brain
  in essential hypertension, 21
  infarction, atherothrombotic, in
    hypertension, 105
Build and Blood Pressure Study: of
  U.S. Society of Actuaries, 105

C

Calcium
  channel blockers, 42
    for hypertension during
      pregnancy, 144
  deficiency, 96
  in pregnancy-induced
    hypertension, 94–96
  relationship to blood pressure, 95
  relationship to magnesium, 95
  restriction
    in preeclampsia-eclampsia,
      151–152
    (in rat), 95
Capillary endothelium, 84
Captopril, 42, 143
Cardiac (see Heart)
Cardiovascular changes
  during hypertension, 70, 103
  during pregnancy, 70
  in pregnancy-induced
    hypertension, 78–80
Cardiovascular disease: family history
  of, 106
Cardiovascular risk factors, 109
Cardiovascular system
  during delivery, 16–17
  during labor, 16–17
Catecholamines, 11
Catheter: Swan-Ganz, 156
Cell(s)
  interstitial, of renal medulla, 58, 67
  juxtaglomerular, 37
  -mediated immunity, 99–100
  responsiveness in preeclampsia,
    100
Cerebral
  blood flow, 79
  intracerebral hemorrhage, 122
  vascular accidents, 105
Cesarean section: in preeclampsia,
  152
Chest radiography, 22
Chlorthalidone, 41
Circulation, 9–12
  adjustments to pregnancy, 13–17
  autoregulation, 9, 11
  hyperdynamic, in preeclampsia, 79

Circulation (cont.)
  regulation of, 9–12
    intrinsic, 9
  uteroplacental regulation,
    kallikrein-kinin system in, 91
Classification: of hypertension, 3–7
Clonidine, 139
Coagulation
  intravascular, 45
    disseminated, 75
  in preeclampsia, 93
  in pregnancy-induced
    hypertension, 93
Coarctation of aorta: and
    hypertension in pregnancy,
    162–163
Cold pressor test, 80
Collaborative Perinatal Project, 113
Colloid osmotic pressure: in
    pregnancy-induced
    hypertension, 134
Complement, 94
Conjunctival vessels: in borderline
    hypertension, 76, 77
Contraception: oral, and renin-
    angiotensin-aldosterone
    system, 86
Contractility: of fibers, 12
Convulsions, 154
Coronary heart disease: in
    hypertension, 105
Corticosteroids, 86
Cortisol: plasma, 86
Cushing's disease, 162
Cytoplasm: endothelial, 84

D

Dahl sensitive and resistant rats, 29
Dehydroisoandrosterone sulfate,
    metabolic clearance, 74
  rate, 75, 165, 168
Delivery
  cardiovascular system during,
    16–17
  in preeclampsia after response to
    therapy, 156
  as therapy for preeclampsia, 131
Dextran: intravenous infusion, 137

Diabetes mellitus
  with diabetic nephropathy, 162
  high blood pressure and, 106
  with secondary hypertension, 163
Diastolic pressure: relationship with
    plasma volume, 27
Diazoxide, 142, 154
  study of, 167
Diet: in hypertension, 134–135
Dihydralazine, 142, 165
Diltiazem, 144
Disseminated intravascular
    coagulation, 75
Diuresis
  osmotic, 152–153
  pressure, 21, 22
Diuretics, 42
  hypertension and, 135–137
  with sympatholytics in severe
    hypertension, 160
  therapy with, 24
  thiazide, 41
    dehydroisoandrosterone sulfate
      and, 165
    in preeclampsia, 152
    during pregnancy, 136
Dopamine
  -beta-hydroxylase, 34
  excretion, 35
Drug(s)
  antihypertensive (see
    Antihypertensive agents)
  anti-inflammatory, nonsteroidal, 57
  for emergencies in hypertension,
    159
  stepped-care approach, 125
  for urgencies in hypertension, 159
Ductus arteriosus: premature closure,
    89

E

Echocardiography, 22
Eclampsia, 3, 5
  blood pressure after, 118, 119
  coagulation in, intravascular, 45
  etiology, 42, 73
  evaluation in, 155–156
  gonadotropin in, chorionic, 88

hypertension prevalence after, 118
  management, 151–156
  in nulliparas, and hypertension,
    117
  recurrent, incidence, 116–117
  survivors, hypertension in, 117
  after treatment, 154
  vascular reactivity in, 80–82
  vasospasm in, 45
  vicious circle of, inner, 78
Edema, 14, 131–132
  during pregnancy, 83
  pulmonary, 26
    acute, 122
Electrocardiography, 21–22
Electrolyte transport: across cell
    membranes, 69
Emergencies, hypertensive, 157–160
  drugs for managing, 159
Enalapril, 42
Endocrine changes
  during hypertension and
    pregnancy, 70
  in pregnancy-induced
    hypertension, 85–88
Endocrine function, 85
Endoperioxides, 45
Endotheliosis: glomerular, 84
Endothelium
  capillary, 84
  cytoplasm, 84
  lesions, glomerular, 75
Endotoxin: and fibrin, 94
Endoxin, 30, 83
Energy-requiring sodium-potassium
    pump, 69
Enzyme(s)
  angiotensin-converting (see
    Angiotensin, -converting
    enzyme)
  converting enzyme inhibitor, 42
  proteolytic, renin and kallikrein as,
    61
Epinephrine: pressor response to,
    80
Equation: Poiseuille, 9
Erythroblastosis fetalis, 163
Erythrocyte: mass changes during
    pregnancy, 14

Essential hypertension, 19–71
  classification, 5
  comparison with pregnancy-
    induced hypertension, 71
  damage to target organs during, 7
  etiologic considerations, 19–71
  mild, 21
  moderate, 21
  pathogenesis, 58
  pathophysiologic subdivisions,
    147–149
  severe, 21
  in sodium-sensitive individuals,
    development of hypertension,
    31
  in women, black and white, study
    of, 58
17-β-Estradiol, 85
Estriol, 85
Estrogens, 13, 163
  secretion in preeclampsia, 88
Estrone, 85
Exercise: regular, in mild
    hypertension, 111
Extracellular fluid
  compartments and
    pathophysiologic subdivisions
    of essential hypertension, 147
  volume
    kidney in, 53
    thiazides and, 135

F

Factors
  VII, VIII, X, XIII, during
    pregnancy, 93
  VIII, consumption in preeclampsia,
    93
Feedback loop: of renin-angiotensin-
    aldosterone, 39
Fetal
  antigen, maternal recognition of,
    98
  growth retardation, 140
  -maternal immunity, 100
  mortality, and high blood pressure,
    114

Fibrin
  degradation products in
    preeclampsia, 93
  deposits in eclampsia, 93
Fibrinogen: during pregnancy, 93
Fibrinolytic system: in pregnancy-
    induced hypertension, 93
Framingham, Massachusetts:
    cardiovascular morbidity and
    mortality study of, 105
Furosemide, 56, 154
  dehydroisoandrosterone sulfate
    and, 165

G

Genetic predisposition: to
    hypertension, 68–69
Glomerular
  endothelial lesions, 75
  endotheliosis, 84
  filtration fraction, 84
  filtration rate, 82, 83, 84, 132
  lesion in preeclampsia, 83
Glomeruloendotheliosis, 4
Glomerulonephritis, 162
Gonadotropin, chorionic, 86
  in eclampsia, 88
Growth
  hormone-prolactin, 86
  retardation, fetal, 140
Guanabenz, 139
Guanadrel, 140
Guanethidine, 140

H

Heart
  (See also Cardiovascular)
  disease
    coronary, in hypertension, 105
    hypertensive, 106
  in essential hypertension, 21
  failure, congestive, in
    hypertension, 105
  hypertrophy, 21
  index, 26
  output, 11
    in borderline hypertension, 21

  in essential hypertension, 19
  increase after hydralazine, 142
  during pregnancy, 15
  in pregnancy-induced
    hypertension, 78–79
  after propranolol, 141
  prostaglandins and, 44
  thiazides and, 135
  rate, 11, 16
    in borderline hypertension, 21
    after diazoxide, 167
    prostaglandins and, 44
  size, effect of sodium intake on,
    32
  sodium and kidney, 26–33
  sounds, fourth, 22
Helminths: and preeclampsia, 96–97
Hemodialysis, 104
Hemodynamic status: and essential
    hypertension pathophysiologic
    subdivisions, 147
Hemodynamics: of hypertension,
    19–26
Hemorrhage: intracerebral, 122
Hemostasis: in pregnancy-induced
    hypertension, 93–94
Histamine, 11
Hormone(s)
  antidiuretic, 29
    prostaglandins and, 45
  growth hormone-prolactin, 86
  melanocyte-stimulating, 86
  sodium-retaining, and kallikrein
    excretion, 60
  suppressor activity in
    preeclampsia, 100
  thyroid-stimulating, 86
  vasoactive, interactions with
    prostaglandins, 50–51
Hydatoxi luaba, 96
Hydralazine, 141, 166
  dehydroisoandrosterone sulfate
    and, 165
  parenteral, 154
Hydrochlorothiazide: and
    dehydroisoandrosterone
    sulfate, 168
9-Hydroxy prostaglandin
    dehydrogenase, 53

Hypercholesterolemia: and high
    blood pressure, 106
Hypertension
  accelerated, 107
  activity and, 127–131
  antihypertensive management (see
      Antihypertensive
      management)
  antihypertensive therapy (see
      Antihypertensive therapy)
  "borderline," 19
    conjunctival vessels in, 76, 77
  chronic, 5
    preeclampsia superimposed on,
      3, 5
    treated women with, perinatal
      outcome in, 115
    in women, perinatal mortality in,
      115
  classification, 3–7
  crisis in, 157
    clinical characteristics of, 158
  Detection and Follow-up Program,
      109
  diagnosis, 4
  diet in, 134–135
  diuretic agents and, 135–137
  eclampsia in nulliparas and, 117
  in eclampsia survivors, 117
  emergencies in, 157–160
    drugs for managing, 159
  essential (see Essential
      hypertension)
  evaluation of, initial, 124
  genetic predisposition to, 68–69
  hemodynamics of, 19–26
  high-renin, 40
  Joint National Commission on
      Detection, Evaluation and
      Management of, 121
  kallikrein-kinin system in, 61–67
  "labile," 19
  late, 5, 163
  low-renin, 39, 40
  malignant, 104, 107
  membrane transport and, 68–71
  mild
    exercise in, regular, 111
    salt restriction in, 111

    therapy, Australian trial, 110
    weight reduction in, 111
  mineralocorticoid-induced, 64
  myocardial function effected by, 28
  plasma and (see Plasma)
  in preeclampsia survivors, 117
  in pregnancy
    classification, 5
    natural history,
        interrelationships, 4
  pregnancy-induced (see Pregnancy-
      induced hypertension)
  prevalence (see Prevalence of
      hypertension)
  renal parenchymal, 67
  renovascular, 42
  secondary
    to adrenal disease, 162
    classification, 5
    to coarctation of aorta, 162
    diabetes and, 163
    to hypoplasia of aorta, 163
    pregnancy and, 161–163
    to renal disease, 161–162
    screening tests for, 124
  severe
    sympatholytic-diuretic therapy,
        160
    vasodilators in, 158
  "transient," 5, 163
  treatment, stepped-care, 110
  types of, 6–7
  urgencies in, 157–160
    drugs for managing, 159
  vasoconstrictor-dependent, 40
  volume-dependent, 40
  volume problem, 131–134
Hypertensive diseases: renin activity
    in, 148
Hypertensive heart disease, 106
Hypertensive pregnancy (see
    Pregnancy-induced
    hypertension)
Hypertensive vascular disease: causes
    and results, 104
Hypertrophy
  heart, 21
  ventricle in, 21
Hypoglycemia, 140

Hypomagnesemia, 95
Hypoplasia: of aorta, 163

I

Ig (*see* Immunoglobulin)
Immune
  complexes, 98–99
  response
    blocking antibody insufficiency
      in preeclampsia, 97
    preeclampsia and, 97–101
    system in preeclampsia, 94
Immunity
  cell-mediated, 99–100
  maternal-fetal, 100
Immunoglobulins, 94
  G, 99
Index: cardiac, 26
Indomethacin, 45, 47, 48
  angiotensin II and, 91
  decreasing renin activity, 56
  inhibiting cyclooxygenase activity,
    52
  prostaglandin cyclooxygenase
    reaction and, 57
  reducing PGE_2 excretion, 58–59
Infarction: atherothrombotic brain, in
  hypertension, 105
Insulin, 79
Interstitial
  cells of renal medulla, 58, 67
  fluid volume, 23
Intracerebral hemorrhage, 122
Intravascular volume, 12, 22

J

Joint National Commission on
  Detection, Evaluation and
  Management of Hypertension,
  121
Juxtaglomerular cells, 37

K

Kallikrein: concentration decrease in
  blacks, 63

Kallikrein-kinin system
  comparison with renin-angiotensin-
    aldosterone system, 62
  deficiency, 63
  in hypertension, 61–67
  interrelationships with renin-
    angiotensin-aldosterone
    system, 61
  in pregnancy-induced
    hypertension, 89–92
  prostaglandins and, 42–67
    interrelationships, 59–61
  in uteroplacental circulation
    regulation, 91
6-Keto-prostaglandin $F_{1\alpha}$, 49
Kidney
  arterial stenosis, renal, 63
  blood flow, 44, 49, 61, 82
  changes
    during hypertension and
      pregnancy, 70
    in pregnancy-induced
      hypertension, 82–85
  damage, 104
  disease
    chronic, 4
    hypertension secondary to,
      161–162
    parenchymal, 23–24, 27, 162
  in essential hypertension, 21
  failure, acute, 162
  function
    changes during pregnancy, 82
    posture and, 83
  involvement in periarteritis
    nodosa, 162
  mass, reduction of, 27
  medulla, interstitial cells of, 58,
    67
  medullary tissues elaborating
    lipids, 67
  parenchymal hypertension, 67
  plasma flow, 82, 84
  polycystic, 162
  pressor system, 42
  prostaglandin metabolism, 44
  prostaglandins and, 53–55
  sodium and heart, 26–33
  tubules, collecting, 58

vascular lesions, 38
vessels (*see* Renovascular)
Kinin
  intrarenal levels, 64
  -kallikrein system (*see* Kallikrein-
    kinin system)
  metabolism, compartmentalization
    of, 65
  -prostaglandin interaction in
    nephron, 66
Kininase(s), 59
  II, 61

L

Labetalol, 140, 165
Labor
  cardiovascular system during,
    16–17
  induction in preeclampsia, 152
Law: Ohm's, 9
Lipids
  antihypertensive medullary, 68
    neutral, 68
    polar, 68
  phosphorolipids, pulmonary
    stabilizing, 152
  vasodepressor, 67–68
Lisinopril, 42
Lithium-sodium countertransport, 69,
    70
Liver blood flow: in pregnancy-
    induced hypertension, 79
Lung
  (*See also* Pulmonary)
  congestion, 33
Lupus erythematosus, 162
Lymphocyte subsets, 100

M

Macula densa: and renin release
    control, 37
Magnesium
  -deficient diet, 95
  in pregnancy-induced
    hypertension, 94–96
  sulfate, 94, 152

Maternal
  antibodies against fetal antigens, 98
  -fetal immunity, 100
  recognition of fetal antigen, 98
Melanocyte-stimulating hormone, 86
Membrane transport: and
    hypertension, 68–71
Metanephrine excretion, 34
Methyldopa, 139
Metoprolol, 140
Mineralocorticoid-induced
    hypertension, 64
Minoxidil, 143
Monoclonal antibodies, 100
  anti-T-cell, 100
Mortality
  fetal, and high blood pressure, 114
  perinatal, 113
    women with chronic
      hypertension and, 115
Muscle
  blood flow in pregnancy-induced
    hypertension, 79
  smooth muscle antibodies, 100
  smooth, vascular, 11
Myocardium
  contractility, 44
  function, adverse effects of
    hypertension on, 28

N

National Health Examination Survey
    of the Public Health Service,
    106
Natriuresis
  atrial factor in, 29, 83
  prostaglandins and, 67
  "third factor" to explain, 83
Nephron: prostaglandin-kinin
    interaction in, 66
Nephropathy
  of analgesic abuse, 55
  diabetic, 162
Nephrotic syndrome, 162
Nervous system
  autonomic (*see* Autonomic nervous
    system)

Nervous system (cont.)
  parasympathetic, 10–11
  sympathetic (see Sympathetic
    nervous system)
Newborn: bradycardia of, 140
Nifedipine, 144
Nitroprusside, 142–143, 154
Norepinephrine, 34
  excretion, 34–35
  plasma, concentration, 34
  pressor response to, 80
  release inhibition, 47

O

Ohm's law, 9
Oral contraception: and renin-
    angiotensin-aldosterone
    system, 86
Osmotic diuresis, 152–153
Oxidants, 94
6-Oxo-prostaglandin $F_{1\alpha}$, 53
  during pregnancy, 93
Oxprenolol, 140

P

Para-aminohippuric acid clearance, 79
Parasympathetic nervous system,
    10–11
Periarteritis nodosa: with renal
    involvement, 162
Perinatal
  Collaborative Perinatal Project, 113
  mortality, 113
    women with chronic
      hypertension and, 115
    outcome in treated women with
      chronic hypertension, 115
Peristalsis: ureteral, 82
PG (see Prostaglandins)
Phenytoin, 154
Pheochromocytoma, 162
Phosphorolipids: pulmonary
    stabilizing, 152
Pindolol, 48
Placenta (see Uteroplacental)
Plasma expansion: in hypertension,
    137–139

Plasma volume, 14, 23
  changes during pregnancy, 14
  contraction in preeclampsia, 79
  in hypertension, 133
  during pregnancy, 134
  relationship with diastolic
    pressure, 27
  arterial, 24
  thiazides and, 135
  in third trimester, 134
Plasminogen activator: during
    pregnancy, 93
Platelet(s)
  aggregation, 52
    inhibition, prostacyclin in, 45–46
  counts, 93
  in pregnancy-induced
    hypertension, 93
  prostaglandins and, 45, 50–53
  thromboxane A_2 of, 52
Poiseuille equation, 9
Polycystic kidney, 162
Posture: and kidney function, 83
Potassium
  ATPase, 30
  deficiency, 32
  depletion, kidney in, 53
  serum, concentration, 32
  -sodium (see Sodium, -potassium)
  stimulating aldosterone secretion,
    38
Prazosin, 142
Preeclampsia, 3, 5
  aldosterone in, 87
  antidiuretic factors in, 88
  blood volume in, 133
  circulation in, hyperdynamic, 79
  coagulation in, intravascular, 45
  estrogen secretion in, 88
  etiology, 42, 73
  evaluation in, 155–156
  helminths and, 96–97
  immune response and, 97–101
    blocking antibody insufficiency
      in, 97
  immune system in, 94
  immunologic basis of, 97
  management, 151–156
  pregnanediol in, 88

Preeclampsia (cont.)
  progesterone in, 88
  renin-angiotensin-aldosterone
      system in, 88
  severe, 152
    maternal consequences of, 153
  sodium retention in, 84–85
  superimposed, 116
    on chronic hypertension, 3
    criteria, 3
    on hypertension, chronic, 5
    recurrences, 3
  survivors, hypertension in, 117
  vascular reactivity in, 80–82
  vasospasm in, 45
  vicious circle of, inner, 78
Pregnancy
  antihypertensive agents during,
      precautions, 145, 146
  antihypertensive management
      during, 125–146
  antihypertensive therapy during,
      122
  blood volume changes during, 14
  cardiac output during, 15
  circulatory adjustments to, 13–17
  elevated blood pressure during,
      consequences, 113–120
  ewe study, 165
  hypertension in (see Hypertension
      in pregnancy)
  hypertensive (see Pregnancy-
      induced hypertension)
  -induced hypertension (see below)
  plasma volume changes during, 14
  rabbit study, 165
  red blood cell mass changes
      during, 14
  secondary hypertension and (see
      Hypertension, secondary)
  "toxemia" of, 3
Pregnancy-induced hypertension, 3,
      73–101
  calcium in, 94–96
  cardiovascular changes in, 78–80
  classification, 5
  colloid osmotic pressure in, 134
  comparison with essential
      hypertension, 71
  endocrine changes in, 85–88
  etiologic considerations, 73–101
  hemostasis in, 93–94
  incidence, 3
  kallikrein-kinin system in, 89–92
  magnesium in, 94–96
  pathophysiology, unified working
      hypothesis for, 92
  prognosis, 116–120
  prostaglandins in, 89–92
  renal changes in, 82–85
  in subsequent pregnancies, 117
Pregnanediol: in preeclampsia, 88
Prekallikrein, 59
  activators, 59
Preload, 12
Pressure
  arterial
    after angiotensin-converting
        enzyme blockade, 149
    diastolic, relationship with
        plasma volume, 24
    long-term level analysis, 23
  blood (see Blood, pressure)
  colloid osmotic, in pregnancy-
      induced hypertension, 134
  diastolic, relationship with plasma
      volume, 27
  diuresis, 21, 22
  -flow regression line (in pregnant
      ewe), 166
  pulmonary capillary wedge, 156
  ventricular filling, 156
Prevalence of hypertension, 1
  in blacks, 1
  after eclampsia, 118
  in men, 1
  in U.S. between 1971–1974, 2
  in whites, 1
  in women, 1
Progesterone, 14
  for hypertension during
      pregnancy, 145–146
  levels during pregnancy, 132
  placental secretion of, 85
  in preeclampsia, 88
  secretion, 83
Prolactin, 13
  -growth hormone, 86

Propranolol, 41, 48, 140
  adverse effects, 141
  prostacyclin and, 50
  prostaglandin excretion and, 59
Prostacyclin, 45, 89
  (*See also* prostaglandins, I_2)
  effect on cyclic-AMP, 50
  of vascular tissues, 52
Prostaglandin(s), 11
  cyclooxygenase, inhibition of, 54
  dehydrogenase
    activity, 52
    9-hydroxy, 53
  E during pregnancy, 90
  E_2, 43, 44, 57
    failure to synthesize, 47
    -9-ketoreductase, 65
    urinary, 58
    uterine blood flow and, 89
    uterine vein, 143
    uterus synthesizing, 89
  effects of, 67
  F_2, 43, 44
  $F_{2\alpha}$, 44
  G_2, 52
  H_2, 52
  I_2, 43, 44, 89
    (*See also* Prostacyclin)
    failure to synthesize, 47
    in preeclampsia-eclampsia, 93
    release into circulation after
      synthesis in vessels of lung, 52
  interactions with vasoactive
      hormones, 50–51
  kallikrein-kinin system and, 42–67
    interrelationships, 59–61
  kidney and, 53–55
  -kinin interaction in nephron, 66
  metabolism
    Bartter's syndrome and, 57
    compartmentalization of, 65
    disorders, 42
    renal, 44
  platelets and, 50–53
  in pregnancy-induced
      hypertension, 89–92
  regulation by, local, 67
  renin-angiotensin-aldosterone
      system and, 55–59

  secretion during pregnancy, 90
  synthesis
    blockade of, 49
    vascular, increase, 81
  synthetase complex, in arachidonic
      acid metabolism, 46
  vessels and, 44–50
Protein
  solution, plasma, 152
  thyroid-binding, 86
Proteinuria, 113
Pulmonary
  (*see also* Lung)
  capillary wedge pressure, 156
  edema, 26
    acute, 122
  stabilizing phosphorolipids, 152
  vascular bed, 45
Pyelonephritis, 162

R

Radiography: chest, 22
Red blood cell: mass changes during
      pregnancy, 14
Reflex: baroreceptor, 25
Renal (*see* Kidney)
Renin
  activity
    high, 39
    in hypertensive diseases, 148
    low, 39
    normal, 39
    plasma, 60
    after vasodilators, 158
  -angiotensin-aldosterone feedback
      loop, 39
  -angiotensin-aldosterone system,
      14, 36–42
    comparison with kallikrein-kinin
      system, 62
    essential hypertension and, 147
    interrelationships with kallikrein-
      kinin system, 61
    in preeclampsia, 88
    in pregnancy-induced
      hypertension, 86
    prostaglandins and, 55–59
  high-renin hypertension, 40

Renin (cont.)
  low-renin hypertension, 39, 40
  release, control of, 37
  substrate, 36
    after estrogen administration, 85
Renovascular
  disease, unilateral, 161
  hypertension, 42
  lesions, 38
Reserpine, 140
Resistance
  (*See also under* Vessels)
  definition, 10
  peripheral (*See also* Vessels,
      peripheral, resistance)
  peripheral, total, 26
    during pregnancy, 19

S

Salt
  balance, and kallikrein, 60
  depletion, chronic, 38
  excretion, prostaglandins in, 45
  restriction
    in mild hypertension, 111
    moderate, 26
Saralasin, 42
Schwartzman reaction, 94
Scleroderma, 162
Secondary hypertension (*see*
      Hypertension, secondary)
Sedation, 127
Serotonin, 11, 77
Smoking: and high blood pressure,
      106
Sodium, 14
  aldosterone release inhibition and,
      38
  balance, changes during
      pregnancy, 82
  body, total, 131
  delivery, and macula densa, 37
  endoxin and, 30
  heart size effected by, 32
  high-sodium diet, 30
  -induced volume overload, 33
  intake
    prostaglandins and, 59

  restriction in preeclampsia-
      eclampsia, 151–152
  of 200 mEq, adaptation of
      sodium resistant subjects, 37
  kidney and heart, 26–33
  -lithium countertransport, 69, 70
  nitroprusside, 142–143, 154
  -potassium
    ATPase, 83
    cotransport, 69
    pump, energy-requiring, 69
  restriction
    during pregnancy, 134
    stringent, 26
  -retaining hormones, and kallikrein
      excretion, 60
  retention in preeclampsia, 84–85
  -sensitive individual, 26
    development of chronic essential
        hypertension in, 31
  stroke volume effected by, 32
Sonogram: for fetal evaluation, 152
Sotalol, 140
Sound: fourth, 22
Spironolactone, 41
Stenosis: renal artery, unilateral, 63
Stepped-care therapy, 110, 125
Stretch receptors: of left atrium, 29
Stroke: in hypertension, 105
Stroke volume, 11, 12, 16
  effect of sodium intake on, 32
  prostaglandins and, 44
Swan-Ganz catheter, 156
Sympathetic nervous system
  activity, 33–35
  block of, 139–140
  essential hypertension and,
      pathophysiologic subdivisions,
      147–148
  renin release control and, 37
Sympatholytic-diuretic therapy: of
      severe hypertension, 160
Systolic time intervals, 22

T

Tachyphylaxis: angiotensin, 47
Teprotide, 42, 143, 148

Thiazide
  chronic therapy, 136
  diuretics (*see* Diuretics, thiazide)
Thrombi: formation of, 46
Thromboplastin, 94
Thromboxane, 43
  A_2 of platelets, 52
  B_2, 45
  during pregnancy, 93
Thyroid
  -binding protein, 86
  -stimulating hormone, 86
"Toxemia of pregnancy," 3
Transcortin, 86
Trophoblast
  antigen deposition, 98
  -specific membrane antigen, 98
Tubules: collecting, 58

U

Ureteral peristalsis, 82
Urgencies, hypertensive, 157–160
  drugs for managing, 159
Urine flow, 82
Uteroplacental
  blood flow, 74, 165
    after hydralazine, 142
  circulation regulation, kallikrein-
    kinin system in, 91
  perfusion impairment, 74–78
Uterus
  blood flow (*see under* Blood, flow)
  gravid, blood flow in, 61
  synthesizing prostaglandin E_2, 89
  vein prostaglandins E_2, 143

V

Vanillylmandelic acid excretion, 34
Vasoactive hormones: interactions
    with prostaglandins, 50–51
Vasoconstriction, 30, 45
Vasoconstrictor
  -dependent hypertension, 40
  fibers, 10
Vasodepressor lipids, 67–68
Vasodilating agents, 24

Vasodilation
  prostacyclin in, 45
  by prostaglandins, 67
Vasodilator(s)
  hemodynamic variables after, 158
  in hypertension during pregnancy,
    141–143
  renin activity after, 158
  system, 63
Vasomotor tone, 10
Vasopressin, 11
Vasospasm
  in eclampsia, 45
  in preeclampsia, 45, 93
Vein(s), 9
  tone, 12
  uterine, prostaglandin E_2, 143
Ventricle, 9
  in hypertrophy, 21
  left
    ejection rate, in borderline
      hypertension, 21
    filling pressure, 156
    systolic function in preeclampsia,
      79
Venules, 9
Verapamil, 144
Vessels
  (*See also* Cardiovascular)
  cerebral, accidents, 105
  conjunctival, in borderline
    hypertension, 76, 77
  endothelium of, in pregnancy-
    induced hypertension, 93
  forearm, resistance in borderline
    hypertension, 21
  hypertensive disease
    angiotensin II generation in, 40
    causes and results, 104
  intravascular volume, 12
  peripheral
    in essential hypertension, 21
    resistance, 44
    resistance, blood pressure
      reduction and, 135
    resistance after hydralazine, 142
    resistance after propranolol, 141
    resistance, regulation of, 11
  prostacyclin of, 52

Vessels (cont.)
  prostaglandins and, 44–50
  pulmonary, bed, 45
  reactivity
    Bartter's syndrome and
      prostaglandin metabolism, 57
    in preeclampsia-eclampsia, 80–82
  receptor, and renin release control,
    37
  renal (*see* Renovascular)
  resistance, 43
    elevation, 46
  systemic, resistance, 16
  tone, in vascular resistance, 43
  volume, 22
  wall, and PGI$_2$ production, 58
Veterans Administration Cooperative
    Study of Antihypertensive
    Agents, 107
Volume
  -dependent hypertension, 40
  depletion and high renin activity,
    40
  -expanded state, 132
  overload, in low-renin
    hypertension, 39–40
  problem, implications for therapy,
    131–134

W

Water
  balance
    changes during pregnancy, 82
    kallikrein and, 60
  body, total, 131, 136
  excretion, prostaglandins in, 45
  retention, 14
Weight reduction: in milk
    hypertension, 111
Whites: prevalence of hypertension
    in, 1

X

X-ray: chest, 22